When worsening health fc
early retirement from offic
re-invented herself as a wi
magazine articles. In this, her first non-fiction
book, she tells the story of her progressive
multiple sclerosis and its impact on her life.
Unflinchingly honest, she paints a picture of 21st
Century Britain as it's never been shown before -
from the perspective of Meg's wheelchair, in a
society where many people think of disability
equality as a "done deal". Never whinging, Meg
tells her sometimes painful story with a warm
humour that will leave you with a new view on
life, society and the realities of disability.

A book that will live in your heart long after
you've finished reading.

For further information about Meg's writing, visit:
www.MonSter-Rainbow.co.uk

The MonSter

and the Rainbow

Memoir of a disability

Meg Kingston

Jay Walker Writing

First published in Great Britain 2010
This edition published by Jay Walker Writing, 2010

® and © 2010 Meg Kingston. All rights reserved.

Meg Kingston asserts the moral right to be identified as the author of this work.

No part of this publication may be reproduced, stored in a retrieval system, or transmitted, in any form or by any means, electronic, mechanical, photocopying, recording or otherwise, without the prior written permission of the publishers.

This book is sold subject to the condition that is shall not, by way of trade or otherwise, be lent, re-sold, hired out or otherwise circulated without the publishers prior consent in any form of binding or cover other than that in which it is published and without a similar condition including this condition being imposed on the subsequent purchaser.

A catalogue record for this book is available from the British Library.

ISBN 978-0-9552602-3-0

Printed and bound in the UK by CPI Antony Rowe

This book would not have been possible without the help, support and advice of many wonderful people. My name is printed on the cover, but many more appear in these pages and some are engraved on my heart. Thank you all.

- Introduction ... 11
  - Prologue ... 13
  - One Tuesday in the Office ... 16
  - Terminology ... 20
  - Chasing Rainbows ... 24
- Seeing Red ... 27
  - We're Still Human ... 29
  - Cloak of Invisibility ... 34
  - Churches and Disability ... 35
  - Disability Rights and Wrongs ... 39
  - Disability in Politics ... 42
  - Disabled Facilities – Open to All ... 45
  - Does She Take Sugar? ... 49
  - Kids' Ride! ... 51
  - What Social Life? ... 54
  - Disability Hate Crime ... 58
  - Begging on the Street ... 60
  - What do I Miss Now I'm Disabled? ... 64
- Orange Juice ... 67
  - You Shouldn't Eat That ... 69
  - Save me from Good Intentions! ... 74
  - Eating Out ... 76
  - Spending Pounds to Spend Pennies ... 79
  - Drugs on Trial ... 81
  - Adapt and Survive ... 84
- Custard Yellow ... 89
  - When to Tell ... 91
  - Working Life ... 96
  - Difficulties in Definition ... 101
  - Waist-High in a Grown-up World ... 104
  - Gadgets ... 108
  - Dignity, Privacy and Other Myths ... 112

  Presenting Disabilities 115
  Let's Shake on That 118
  Family Gatherings 120
  Returning to Work 124
  Retiring on Health Grounds 127
Being Green 131
  The Green-Eyed Monster 133
  Disability Etiquette 136
  Vegboxes and Delivery Men 142
  Public Transport 145
  The Power of Thought 151
  Things I Wish Someone Had Told Me 155
  Relearning Skills 158
  Call Me Oracle 161
  Disability v Disability 164
  Doctors – The Manual 167
The Blues 173
  Symptom Poker 175
  Too Tall, Too Short and Possibly Too Fat 177
  Daytime TV and Other Terrors 181
  Drunk and Disorderly - or Disabled 185
  Money Matters 187
  Paranoia 190
  Disability Charities 193
  Accidents and Emergencies 196
My Friend Indigo 201
  Trampering 203
  Prince Philip's Steps 205
  Coping Strategies 209
  Life's Too Short 215
  Two Kinds of Youth 218
  Dear Winner 220
  To Whom it May Concern 223

    Talking Cure 226
    Underground, Overground 229
Violet Elizabeth 231

    You're Disabled - Here's my Problem 233
    A Wheelchair is Public Property 236
    No-one Warned Me 240
    You Look So Well! 242
    What is Accessible? 243
    What is a Symptom? 246
    Trust Me, I'm a Doctor 249
    Boys Don't Make Passes 252
    Blaming the Victim 255
    The Rules of Complaining 257
    The Only Certainty 260

The Rainbow and other happy places 265

    Happy Places 267
    The Printed Word 270
    The Virtual World 273
    Prescribed Exercise and Other Programs 277
    The Write Way 280
    Publish and Don't be Damned 286
    Learning for Life 291
    Local Learning 296

Afterword 301

    And Finally 303

Introduction

Prologue

This is a true book, the events I describe really happened to me. I have taken small liberties by occasionally combining similar events into a single occurrence, but it's all true.

I have, however, concealed the identities of many people and places for several reasons. Firstly, I appreciate that other people may remember events differently, or may not wish to be associated with their previous actions. So rather than spend months trying to track down everyone who gets a mention and ensure they're happy with my comments, I chose not to identify them. If a reader thinks they recognise themselves in this book but don't agree with my telling of the events as they remember them – please understand that this is my memory of how it happened. It's also possible that I'm describing another, similar event or have combined your incident with another one for readability. I do identify some individuals and groups who have made a positive contribution to my experiences of life as a disabled person and to them I offer this book with my gratitude.

When I write, whether it's a short story or a magazine article, I have an "ideal reader" in my mind. Whilst writing this book, I have thought about a very particular reader – myself, as I was all those years ago. In this book, I describe many of the events that took me by surprise when I first encountered them as a person with a disability. It's a serious problem that no-one tells the newly-diagnosed much about the medical aspects of their chronic condition, but even less warning is given about the social implications. Through anecdotes and my commentary, I've set out to provide a guide to life as a disabled person in the early 21st Century. I hope my experiences will be valuable to those with different chronic illnesses and in other situations, as well as fellow MS sufferers. I've discussed many of these events with people who have other conditions, and found that we all have very similar experiences. I have also counselled several newly-diagnosed people (most with MS, but not all) and their input has shaped the way I talk about many of my own experiences. To all of these people, who did not know their comments were contributing to my writing this book, I extend my gratitude. Any misunderstandings in here are, of course, entirely my own.

Why the MonSter?

When I came across the use of the word MonSter as slang for MS, I felt that someone had found the perfect name for the condition. Capitalising the M and the S works well and believe me – MS *is* a monster. There are times when I could almost believe it's a separate, malevolent presence that has more control over my body than I do. There have been times when I've rested for days, ready to go somewhere important, only to have my MS suddenly decide I won't have any energy after all. When I suffer from intention tremors and strange, inexplicable symptoms, I can almost hear my MonSter laughing at me as it pulls my strings like a puppet-master.

People who suffer from cancer are sometimes advised to think of the growth as a separate "thing" inside their body and to hate that lump; rather than feeling it to be part of themselves. It's similar with my MonSter. By thinking of it as a separate, self-willed entity, I detach it from myself and remember that I do have an existence apart from my disability.

Why the Rainbow?

As soon as I started writing this book, I realised that it was going to have a lot of very short chapters, which don't follow any particular order. For convenience, I wanted to group similar topics together and came up with the idea of using the colours of the rainbow as headings for these groups. So I could put a lot of things that make me angry under "Seeing Red"; those connected with food under "Orange Juice", and so on. The groupings may be arbitrary, but it breaks the chapters up neatly.

I also wanted to use the positive associations of the rainbow against the negative image of the MonSter. Whether we see a rainbow as a symbol of God's promise, a signpost to a pot of gold or a manifestation of the laws of physics, I think we can all agree on its beauty. There are beautiful and positive aspects to disability, as well as the MonStrous and negative ones.

One Tuesday in the Office

29 years old with a husband, a stable job and plans for the future, I went into the office like anyone else that morning, and left as a disabled person, although I didn't know it, at the end of the day.

I worked for the IT Department of a local council, involving long hours of technical work and being available out-of-hours on a rota. I'd been doing similar work for years in different places and loved the work. Well, most of it.

This particular Tuesday started at eight o'clock in the office. I had a few odd tingles in my legs in the morning, but assumed I'd been sitting awkwardly. At lunchtime, I wandered round the shops but my low-heeled court shoes kept slipping off as I walked. At one point my legs buckled, and I grabbed a lamppost for support. An elderly lady came to my assistance, much to my embarrassment, and I chose to retreat to the office. It amazes me now that I didn't think about the strange events all afternoon and it never crossed my mind that something was seriously wrong. At the end of the day, I stood up to leave the desk, and had to grab at furniture to stop myself falling over. My legs were oddly numb and weak; I couldn't even walk to the door without holding on to something.

I stopped at the Doctor's surgery on my way home, and insisted on seeing my GP The receptionist squeezed me in between his scheduled appointments, but the doctor just dismissed my symptoms. He insisted it was a pinched nerve after the bad back I'd recently suffered from rowing on the River Wear. He prescribed painkillers (which I didn't need) and bed rest (which I didn't want). I had no choice but to go home.

The following morning, the weird numbness in my legs was worse. I dug out an old walking stick I'd used for rambling and took this to work with me. By now, I was seriously concerned but didn't know what to do. The Doctor's practice closed all day Wednesday, and I didn't feel it was serious enough to go to Casualty, so I waited until open surgery on Thursday. Once again the GP assured me nothing was wrong and made it clear he thought I was wasting his time. He offered to sign me off work for a month, citing stress. I refused and kept making appointments every two days, insisting he take my symptoms seriously. After two weeks of these visits, he finally promised to refer me to an orthopaedic specialist. I badgered the details of his proposed referral from the receptionist. Armed with the consultant's name, I called the secretary at his private rooms and she arranged for me to see the consultant after his last appointment in two days' time. I'd have to pay, but at least I was going to see a doctor who might actually listen to me instead of just patting my hand and dismissing my complaints.

On Thursday afternoon, I arrived early and settled in the waiting area. The consultant listened to my symptoms, prompting me occasionally and asking questions. He examined me in a way I'd never experienced before, but I now know to be a standard, basic neurological examination. Then we talked.

"I want you to come into hospital for further tests," he began.

"I'm sorry," I said. "I can't afford to pay for tests. I only paid for this consultation because I didn't want to wait months for an appointment on the NHS."

"It's alright," he replied. "I'll get you into the NHS hospital. If your GP had told me how severe your symptoms were, I'd have seen you just as quickly with an NHS referral." He didn't waive his fee, though.

The following day, a Friday, I was admitted to the NHS hospital for tests. A week later they transferred me to a specialist neurological team at another hospital. After a fortnight of tests, I was sent home without a diagnosis. Some tests had proved negative, some were inconclusive, but none was positive. The neurological team had detailed evidence of my problems, visible and invisible, but I had no firm diagnosis. I was told to take things easy, avoid stressful situations and come back in three months for a progress check. The neurologist told me there was no need for me to take time off work, but I should do so if I felt it would help. Acutely aware that I'd already taken a considerable amount of sick leave, my walking stick and I were back in the office the next day.

This pattern continued for a couple of years. My symptoms stabilised. The three-monthly neurological checkups became six-monthly and lasted less than three minutes a time. The management at work treated me with suspicion and some friends made excuses not to meet up. My life had changed, but I was learning to live with the changes. My husband was supportive, taking over chores that had become difficult for me and refusing to be ruffled by the changes in our lives.

August, a Few Years Later

My routine visits to the neurologist followed a pattern: I'd describe any new symptoms I thought might be relevant and was sent home with nothing more than a few platitudes. At this particular appointment, I described my new symptoms – tingling and a lack of control of my left hand. The neurologist asked if I could cope with it.

"Sort of," I said. "I can't knit because of it, but I manage most things."

"Well, even if it is MS ..." he replied.

I didn't even hear the rest of the sentence. My stomach had dropped through the floor and my brain had shut down.

"Pardon?"

"It's quite possible it's multiple sclerosis, but we can't do anything to help either way," he said.

"But you told me the test was negative," I knew they'd tested for MS as one of the first possibilities.

"We don't have a proper test for MS," he answered, checking his watch. "A negative doesn't mean you haven't got it, just that it doesn't show on the test."

He ended the appointment, insisting he didn't have time to elaborate further. I hit the library, looked up MS and recognised other symptoms I hadn't guessed were connected. I knew now that I was disabled!

Several years later, I read my medical records and found that the doctors had "strongly suspected" it was MS from the start. There's no explanation for their not telling me earlier. This wasn't uncommon practice at the time, and the only defence I've ever heard was that they might have been reluctant to give me a diagnosis of something they couldn't treat. Whatever the reasons, I'm pleased to know this happens much less often now, largely due to the availability of information on the internet and the ready availability of MRI scanners.

Terminology

I use some unusual words in this book that may not be known to every reader – a mixture of medical terms and slang. Here's a list, with a brief (not always serious) description for each one.

Acronym   An abbreviation, usually of a medical term. Half of the entries in this list are acronyms!

Atrophy   Medical term that describes the way muscles shrink if they aren't used.

BSL   British Sign Language. A means of communication for people with limited hearing or speaking abilities. It's worth everyone learning the alphabet in their local sign language, just in case. Watching a practiced Signer is truly impressive – it's almost like dancing.

CNS   Central Nervous System. The brain and spinal cord– the parts of the body primarily affected by MS.

DABDA   The five stages of coping with tragedy or grief, invented by Elisabeth Kübler-Ross in 1969: Denial, Anger, Bargaining, Depression, Acceptance.

DDA   Disability Discrimination Act (1995). The main law in the British legal system that forbids discrimination against people on grounds of their disability. Allegedly.

DMD   Disease Modifying Drug, as opposed to drugs intended to treat specific symptoms.

GP   General Practitioner. In countries other than the UK, this is sometimes called a "family doctor".

Hug   A truly misnamed symptom, the "MS Hug" can be anything from a mild tingling to a crushing pain that lasts for days, even weeks. It can be felt anywhere from the waist to the shoulders and doesn't have to be a full "hug" – can just be one patch. Caused by small muscles (usually the intercostals) going into spasm.

Icky   Slang term for slightly distasteful. Not quite disgusting, and not gory, either.

Intention Tremors   An inexplicable trembling of part of the body when trying to move it. Often affects hands and eyes.

Jelly Belly   Slang term for a common condition amongst wheelchair users, referring to the loss of stomach muscle tone.

ME   Myalgic Encephalomyelitis. Also known as Yuppie Flu or Chronic Fatigue Syndrome. A condition which is sometimes confused with MS, mainly due to the similar acronym.

MS   Multiple Sclerosis. A disease of the CNS which is the commonest neurological disorder amongst adults in the Western world. The Latin term means "many scars", referring to the lesions the condition causes on the brain and spinal cord.

MonSter   Slang term for MS when spelt with capitalised "M" and "S", sometimes edited out by spellcheckers.

MSer   Slang term for a person who has Multiple Sclerosis. Pronounced "Em-esser". The plural is "MSers".

Myelin Medical term for the fatty, protective layer that protects the nerves in the spine. Picture it as the insulation around a mains wire.

NHS   National Health Service. The UK's state-funded healthcare provider.

OT   Occupational Therapist. Someone qualified to assess both a person's abilities and what can be done to make life easier for them. A good OT is worth their weight in helpful gadgets!

Placebo   A "sugar pill" given to patients in double-blind trials, so they (and the doctor) don't know whether they are getting the actual drug or not.

Placebo effect Medical term which refers to the way patients get better even if they aren't on the real drug. A powerful demonstration of the ability of the human mind to improve the condition of the body.

PPMS Primary Progressive MS. A label given to someone who has confirmed MS but has never had a remission – their condition just gets progressively worse.

RADAR   The Royal Association for Disability and Rehabilitation – they operate a National Key Scheme for accessible public toilets.

Relapse   Medical term for a period when MS symptoms get worse.

Remission   Medical term for a period when a person's MS symptoms improve.

RRMS Relapsing-Remitting MS. The commonest form of MS and the diagnosis everyone is given at first. Their condition is characterised by a series of bad episodes (relapses) and improvements (remissions).

RRP   Recommended Retail Price. Quoted by the manufacturer of a product, but not necessarily what is charged by a retailer.

SATOFSAT   Sick And Tired Of Feeling Sick And Tired. My usual response to the question, "How are you **really** feeling?"

SPMS Secondary Progressive MS. A debatable label, as definitions vary. Roughly, it's given to someone who has confirmed MS and either has only minor remissions or started with the relapsing-remitting form but has stopped having remissions – their condition now gets progressively worse.

Wheelie   Slang term for wheelchair user.

Chasing Rainbows

"Miracle Cure for Multiple Sclerosis."
"Eating Bananas Cured my MS."
"My Mother Wished her MS Away."

Okay, I made those up. But similar headlines appear in the press on a regular basis. It's a particular problem with something like MS, because symptoms can improve suddenly and people tend to associate that improvement with what they were doing at the time. So if you've been eating a lot of bananas lately and your MS goes into remission, it's easy to conclude it's the bananas that did it. Maybe they did. But it's probably just a coincidence.

After years of seeing claims like these reported in the press, I've grown very sceptical about anything hailed as a cure. Someday, one will be found and it's likely to be something unexpected. But I'll wait for a good success rate in trials before I get excited about it. I know plenty of people with all sorts of chronic conditions who pursue every rumour of a treatment – the wackier the better. While I understand their wishing to be healthy again, it's foolish to disregard the risks. I wince when I hear of people getting experimental surgery or buying unlicensed drugs off the internet. Maybe it'll help, *maybe* it won't hurt – but doctors in the 1950s thought Thalidomide was harmless for pregnant women.

Another aspect to this is that friends give me press cuttings of the latest rumour. The media, of course, never talk about the low success rate and sweep any unfortunate ill effects under the metaphorical carpet. You'd never sell any papers with a headline like: "1 in 5 MS Sufferers May be Helped by Radical Surgery (If It Doesn't Make Them Worse!)" and truth is not the highest priority when writing for newspapers. I know – I've done it. It's very difficult to explain this to someone who thinks I should be over the moon to hear that an MSer has apparently been cured by an ancient Egyptian ceremony. I try to be gracious, but I'm unlikely to do more than research the claimed cure on the internet. Sometimes I keep an eye on developments, but these miracle treatments usually vanish as quickly as they appear.

If someone's chronic condition suddenly gets better, then I'm happy for them. If they attribute this to a "cure", I smile politely and wish them well. If the same results can be repeated in other patients without ill effects, then I'll start to pay attention. I've had experimental treatments for my MS, but only under carefully controlled conditions, with medical staff on-hand to deal with any possible problems. There's a big difference between clinical trials and buying something over the internet to inject into your own body.

A further problem with "cures" that people are unwilling to discuss is that alleviating the original problem doesn't miraculously wind the clock back. After all these years of enforced immobility, I know nothing is going to restore my ability to walk 40 miles in a day. (I did plenty of sponsored walks in my pre-MonSter days.) The secondary effects of a chronic condition can be even more debilitating than the disease itself and much harder to cure.

One of the difficulties with MS – and many other illnesses – is that no-one really knows what causes it. I have a suspicion that two or more different illnesses are diagnosed as MS, which could explain why some of us respond to a treatment and others not at all. At the time of writing, there is a surgical operation being hailed as the cure for MS. But even its inventor says it's only suitable for about half of the MS patients he scans. Maybe it will be the answer, at least for some of us, but I'll wait for the procedure to be peer-reviewed and proper clinical assessments made before I consider it.

Hopefully there will come a day when we not only know what causes the MonSter but can successfully treat 100% of cases. Maybe we'll achieve a Utopia where no-one needs suffer *any* ailment, disability or illness. I doubt I'll live to see it, though. In the meantime, I will focus my energy on fighting my MonSter's secondary effects rather than waiting for a miracle to banish him.

Seeing Red

We're Still Human

From Dickens's times the media have portrayed disabled people in two categories. Either we're sufferers - terribly noble but ultimately doomed; or we're obsessive megalomaniacs with dire plans for the future of society.

My problem is – I'm neither as noble as Tiny Tim nor as evil as a Bond baddie.

Every day, people's behaviour demonstrates similar views. I'm not sure whether the press lead or follow common opinions, I just wish for a better representation of us.

I was shopping for special treats in Marks & Spencer Food Hall. In my wheelchair, I balanced the basket on my lap and had already sought assistance from friendly shoppers who'd been happy to pass me items I couldn't reach.

A lady approached me, making eye contact and smiling widely. I assumed she was about to offer to help and smiled back. To my surprise, she simply said,

"I think you're wonderful."

"I'm sorry?" I replied, trying to work out where she knew me from and what I might have done that she appreciated so much.

"You're in a wheelchair – I think all people in wheelchairs are absolutely wonderful," she explained and continued to beam, waiting for my reply.

I'm not one to give insincere thanks, and I could hardly tell her I found her remark ridiculous. I considered being very rude; but in the end I just replied,

"Good for you."

She looked surprised at this response (probably due to my terse manner) and said nothing further as I wheeled away.

I'm sure she thought she was being nice, but such comments are patronising. There's no more reason people in wheelchairs should conform to a single stereotype than all pensioners, redheads or everyone over six feet tall. We certainly don't all appreciate such inexplicable comments from strangers. But the media has often encouraged this view that somehow being in a wheelchair defines everything about a person's character.

Things are improving slowly. Increasingly, we are portrayed as normal people who just happen to have a disability. The BBC series *Beyond Boundaries* is a fantastic example of disabled people being shown, warts and all, in situations that would be difficult for anyone. In overcoming tremendous obstacles, the various participants show their true colours. Participants may be bad-tempered shouters, stoical triers, moaning minnies or even prima donnas; the important thing is that they all come across as **human**. It's a shame that we've needed programmes to feature disabled people exclusively to get this shown on television, although a small number have finally begun to appear in magazine and reality shows.

A large number of disabled characters are still played by able-bodied actors, a practice commonly known as "blacking-up" in reference to the now-unacceptable custom of white actors being made-up to play non-white characters, such as Laurence Olivier playing Othello[1]. This may have been acceptable for programmes such as

---

[1] The phrase "blacking up" has been used in this context in many different places. Several people, some disabled, some not, claim to be the originator. I believe they have each invented it independently, rather than copying it. The only thing I can say for sure about its first use is, "It wasn't me!"

Ironside, but less so nowadays. Some programmes feature an able-bodied comedian faking incontinence or jumping out of a wheelchair for laughs. I know many people (including some with disabilities) find this entertaining, but I'm not one of them. I enjoy humour that laughs along with disabled people about their disability, but not where disabilities make people easy targets for cheap gags. As someone who uses a wheelchair some of the time, but not always, I'm frequently annoyed by people telling me I only use the wheelchair because I'm lazy, or thinking it's funny to joke about me leaping out of it and running around. Trust me – pushing yourself about in a manual wheelchair is not an easy option, but it's safer than trying to walk when your legs won't co-operate.

People with disabilities are sometimes cast in roles that would be impossible for someone without their impairments; from short people in films like "Time Bandits" to amputees appearing in "Spartacus" (although these battle scenes have allegedly been cut from the movie for being too realistically gory). Thankfully, there has been a steady increase in actors playing characters who have the same impairment as the actor themselves. I can think of "Four Weddings and a Funeral", "The Office", "The Secret Diary of a Call Girl", "Everytime You Look at Me" and now Eastenders. I know the BBC now have a policy to always use an actor with the same disability as the one they're playing and hope this trend will continue.

Freak-show television is still a reality in the 21st Century. Although it's portrayed as sympathetic, I find the programmes focussing on deformity distasteful. I see this genre as anti-equality, as it encourages the opinion that it's acceptable to treat someone who's different as an object, rather than a person.

Not everyone welcomes the idea of disabled people being visible in this way. In early 2009, Cerrie Burnell joined CBeebies as a presenter and complaints from parents began to arrive. Interestingly, TV reports of the situation were presented in such a way that I knew she was disabled and that parents claimed she was scaring their children – but the reports didn't mention anything about her disability. I had to search on the internet to find she was born with her right arm ending just below her elbow. All credit to her, the BBC and everyone involved for keeping her in the job and not giving in to the controversy over a visibly disabled person working in a role that could be done by an able-bodied actor!

Obviously, it's difficult to cast a disabled actor for a role in which they're disabled for part of the plot, able-bodied for the rest. Hence films like "Hilary and Jackie" (about the life of MS sufferer Jacqueline du Pre) and "Go Now" (about a healthy young man who develops MS) have to cast able-bodied people in the lead roles. Each of these films portrays the changes wrought by MS realistically, with impressive acting by the leads in both. I've never heard of such a role being played by a disabled actor where the production team has to find ways to portray them as able-bodied – but it might happen! I'm told there is an Australian soap opera where regular characters are prone to developing disabilities, chronic health problems and even terminal illnesses, before being miraculously cured. People have suggested we should all move to Australia where something in the air can cure anything!

The overriding reason for a person appearing with a disability (real or simulated) in any creative work tends to be *because* of their disability. This is changing – at least with respect to extras. It's increasingly likely that a crowd scene will include at least one person with a visible disability (one of the zombies in "Shaun of the Dead" is a wheelchair user). This equality has yet to reach the level of leading actors, where any significant disability disqualifies an applicant; but that, too, will change with time. The day will come when someone might be cast in a role that doesn't rely on their disability, just as an actor can play a role that isn't defined by the colour of his skin.

Cloak of Invisibility

Beloved of boy wizard fans the world over, few people realise that cloaks of invisibility really exist. I'm as noticeable as anyone, but I can slip into my cloak and suddenly – you can't see me! I'm not joking. Here are some comments from members of the public, once I've made myself conspicuous by speaking to them:

"I didn't realise anyone else was in the queue."

"Oh, is it your shopping? I thought someone had just left it here."

"Shouldn't you have a flag or something? So people can see you coming."

Okay, so it's a wheelchair, not really an invisibility cloak. But it works. All of those comments (and many more) are genuine – people just can't see someone sitting in a wheelchair. I've had someone pick up the basket of shopping I'd laid on the floor, taking it away because there was no-one nearby. I'm sat next to it, reaching for something on the shelf, but I'm invisible!

So why don't they see me? I'm not a small person by any means. I dress in bright colours; I'm likely to be wearing a hat and the frame of my wheelchair is purple.

Perhaps it's a height thing; am I beneath their radar because I'm only waist-high? But wouldn't that make children invisible, too? Adults certainly notice kids.

Is it embarrassment? Is dealing with a wheelchair user so difficult that their brains screen out the discomforting sight? Do they think I'll vanish if they pretend I'm not there?

No, I don't know the answer. Perhaps we should run an ad campaign – like reminding drivers to look out for motorbikes.

Think adult, think child, think wheelchair!

Churches and Disability

Faced with an uncertain future, many people with chronic illnesses turn to their religion for comfort and support. I'm sure some of them find it.

Several years ago, I contacted our then-nearest church. I wanted to warn them someone on crutches planned to attend and ask if they had any preferences about where I sat, to avoid my crutches being in anyone's way. I also wondered if they would prefer me to arrive early for a service. The answer surprised me.

"We'd rather you didn't," he said.

"Sorry? Didn't arrive early? Would it be better to come at the last minute?"

"We'd rather you didn't bring crutches into our church. They'd scratch the floor."

At least he was being honest with me.

"The floor?"

"It's parquet and it was very expensive." He'd started talking slowly, as if I might not understand him.

"That's no problem. The rubber ferrules stop them scratching floors."

"Those things are even worse – they leave terrible marks."

"Would it be better if I came in my wheelchair?"

"Has it got tyres on it? They're just as bad."

I can take a hint. That church values their new floor above my possible attendance - and I don't like people who hide behind the word "we" to express their own opinions. Ironically, I'd already been in there several times– it was our local polling station and no-one had ever told me I couldn't vote on crutches.

I phoned another local-ish church and left a message. Someone called me back but didn't identify himself.

"Are you the handicapped woman asking about wheelchair access?"

"I'm the disabled person who left a message about ramped access to your church, yes. Is there a door round the back I can use or something?"

"No, there isn't. We don't offer special treatment for people like you. We expect our congregation to make the effort."

"To make what effort?" I asked, not quite believing what he'd said.

"It's symbolic, you see. You're entering a higher place. It wouldn't be appropriate to make it easy."

"I'm sorry – are you saying that people can only get into heaven if they can climb stairs?"

"Don't be stupid. It's a metaphor – look the word up if you don't understand."

I took a deep breath. "I understand metaphors – but you seem to be saying your church is only open to those who can get up the steps."

"Look," he sounded annoyed now. "There's no point calling me up and insisting you have special rights. And you can't sue us – churches are exempt from the DBA."

He hung up.

I was fairly sure he meant the DDA, but I wasn't about to call back, correct his acronym and explain that churches aren't exempt.

Some months later, he rang again, but still didn't give me his name.

"Is this the woman who complained we had to provide a ramp into our church?"

"Erm, I don't think that's quite what I would have said. Which church are you talking about?"

He told me and continued, "We've applied for a lottery grant and they've said they'll pay half the money if we raise the other half."

"That's great," I said. "Well done."

"So you'll pay half?" he asked.

I won't document my exact words here, but I made it clear that I didn't want anything to do with a church who expected me to donate half the cost of building a ramp before I could even enter. There was no proper access by the time we moved away from the area – presumably they didn't find anyone else willing to stump up the money, either.

I appreciate the difficulties in making places of worship accessible, but I find some people's attitude very hard to reconcile with their proclaimed faith. Why should a disabled individual pay thousands of pounds to make a public building accessible? Or if a building is already accessible, how can anyone tell me that I'm only welcome if I don't use my crutches or wheelchair? Not what I call a Christian point of view.

Speaking of Christian views, the various faith-based doorsteppers who've rung my doorbell usually have something to say about disability. It's interesting to hear them tell me how I "have more need to repent than most" and quote verses about *the halt and the lame,* or Leviticus 21:18; although they generally (not always!) stop short of saying my disability is some sort of judgement. Then they back-pedal when I ask about accessibility at their particular church. The Christian Union at an office I used to work in said it would be "awkward" to hold their meetings in a ground floor room. I know other people with disabilities who've experienced this attitude of "you really need to go to church – but not ours!"

Most of the churches I've attended have odd ideas about accessibility. I've often wanted to tell them that:
Wheelchairs don't fit through narrow doorways or aisles;
Gravel car parks and certain carpets are really hard work for a wheelchair;
Disabled people don't often bring their own squad of able-bodied helpers;
Not all of us want to sit at the back for the whole service.

Not all religious establishments are so blinkered about disabled people – see page 267 for an example of one that positively welcomes us. I've seen some that are properly accessible, but many more that claim to be, although they've evidently never asked anyone in a wheelchair to check.

Disability Rights and Wrongs

"You can't buy that!" said the grey-haired woman in the supermarket.

"I'm sorry," I replied, putting the pack of pork chops down. "Is there something wrong with it?"

She grabbed the same pack and pushed me to one side so she could look through the reductions fridge.

"This is the pensioners' fridge. You're not supposed to look in here."

An interesting point of view and unenforceable in law, even if the supermarkets were inclined to try. But it's not the only time I've been told I'm not entitled to something because another group of people think they have a monopoly. The usual reason I'm told I can't use a disabled toilet, parking space or whatever is that I'm not old enough. Age is not a disability. Although many elderly people are disabled, the date on a birth certificate isn't what makes someone disabled. Also, the lack of these years does not mean someone is less disabled than an older person.

The UK Disability Discrimination Act of 1995 defines a disabled person thus: *a person has a disability for the purposes of this Act if he has a physical or mental impairment which has a substantial and long-term adverse effect on his ability to carry out normal day-to-day activities.*

The sheer wooliness of this definition reflects the common difficulty in defining something as nebulous as disability. Some questionnaires ask "Do you consider yourself to have a disability?" Instead of labelling someone, they want us to label ourselves. There is no longer a register of disabled people in the UK, (although I do get asked "Are you registered as disabled?"). Any workable definition has to come from a description of what someone is and is not capable of doing. Specifically, it should not include people who just want to call themselves disabled.

I cannot count the number of times I've been told that someone is allowed to use a disabled parking space / toilet because they're pregnant / have a child with them / have sprained their ankle / are delivering something. If someone is sufficiently debilitated by a long-term condition, they can apply for a disabled parking badge – there is no automatic entitlement and using a badged space without displaying the badge is an offence. The law is that simple. As for the "I'm only going to be a second" brigade, don't get me started!

There are few enough facilities for the disabled without them being used by non-disabled people who could use another loo or parking space.

Once, I approached the only disabled loo at the theatre, a little worried by the queue length. As I got closer, I scanned the people waiting, thinking that no-one looked as if they had a disability – which is unusual. Many disabilities don't show, it's true – but if you've got seven people waiting for a disabled loo, I'd expect some of them to have walking sticks, etc. Then I noticed that everyone was staring at posters, the wall, the ceiling – anywhere but in my direction. Finally, as I neared the back of the line, someone coughed and waved me to the front, where I waited until the very fit-looking member of staff came out, muttering something about being in a hurry. At least they all had the decency to make way for the person who genuinely needed an accessible loo – but they wouldn't walk up a dozen steps to use the non-disabled facilities.

Laziness doesn't count as a disability, either.

There's a strong tendency in the UK to focus on disability issues that affect either children or elderly people. Whether it's organised events, charities, publicity or the provision of facilities, disabled adults are frequently disregarded. I've counted stalls at disability events on several occasions and found that less than 10% are aimed at people between the ages of 18 and 60. I can see how this comes about – people are always more interested in helping children than adults and everyone hopes for a long, happy retirement, so we can see the point of supporting pensioners. But what about those of us in the middle? Disabilities don't automatically vanish when you become an adult, only to reappear when you retire.

Disability in Politics

At the time of writing, the UK has just had the most closely-fought General Election in decades. Before deciding how to vote, I had a look at what the various parties said on the subject of disability. This wasn't a major task. In fact, there's been so little mention of the subject that I was beginning to think all disabled people have either become invisible or been miraculously cured.

Pardon my cynicism.

The problem is, there are relatively few disabled people compared to other lobbying groups, such as those who plan to retire some day(!). There's no overall structure to the disabled community, so we don't co-ordinate our votes and we have a higher proportion of non-voters than most groups. In other words, we don't have much political clout and we're assumed to cost more public money than able-bodied people. So the parties tend to ignore us.

I've scoured the leaflets pushed through our letter box by various parties, looking for mention of disabled people or policies to improve access. Not one word. One of our local parties regularly asks residents to let them know their concerns and I have returned the forms several times, asking that they address our inaccessible railway station and similar matters. I've never had a reply, although I've heard that they are finally looking into these problems.

Local councillors have been a little more helpful. I was recently contacted by a member of our Town Council, asking for my help in assessing planned changes to local footpaths. She's hoping they can improve facilities for those of us with electric buggies, without too much expense. Well, it's worth a try and I did survey the site in question and let her know my findings. Interestingly, she had approached a local disability group for just such input, but didn't get an answer.

I appeared on the front page of our local paper in after the council elections of 2008. I'd gone to our polling station and made my way to the lift, only to find it was closed for refurbishment. When asked, the staff said it had been for some months and it would be for several more. I had to struggle down the stairs on my crutches, with my husband trying to prevent anyone else from jostling me as they hurried past. I checked the website where details of all polling stations are available, which stated that a lift was available. I phoned the council, but they didn't want to know. So I sent my story to the local paper. They contacted the council, who replied that there is level access available, by going around the outside of the building and knocking on the fire door so that one of the polling staff can open it. It's several hundred yards, there were no signs and the staff I spoke to were unaware of this route. The council officially apologised for any inconvenience caused.

Disenfranchising people who can't manage stairs is just an inconvenience?

I'm pleased to report that the lift was working for the recent general election – and there were plenty of signs indicating the route for mobility-impaired voters. Hopefully, everyone got to vote this time.

I did check the online manifestoes of all the major parties and was disappointed to see how little they mentioned disability. One party promised financial backing to help disabled people into politics at a local level, but it wasn't a lot of money to cover the whole country.

Some organisations try to politicise disabled people, but never in a way I can relate to. I think disability *must* be discussed in the political arena and that disabled people should be involved in government at all levels. But it's also important to have something to say on other issues. I wouldn't vote for someone whose only political statement was, "Vote for me – I'm disabled", any more than I would vote for any other single-policy party.

There have been a few politicians with disabilities. Our recently-deposed Prime Minister was unsighted in one eye and there was one MP who was completely blind. I should also mention that several prominent ministers have children with disabilities. But that's a much smaller proportion than disabled people form in the population as a whole. I'm sure it's partly because disabled people often don't have the energy to take part in politics, as well as accessibility issues.

Will able-bodied people vote for a disabled person? Obviously it does happen, but in my own experience, many people assume that someone with a disability is incapable of achieving anything an able-bodied person could do. Yes, there would be a few sympathy voters, but I think they'd be outnumbered by the ones who think we're ineffective or that we're incapable of having any interest in issues other than disability.

So what is the solution? I believe there should be people with disabilities in all parts of society, including politics. I welcome the idea that our newly-elected government is promising to encourage this, but there are more problems that need to be addressed. Some Town Halls and other council buildings are not accessible, so it would be impossible for a mobility-impaired person to carry out the usual duties of a politician. If disabled voters can't even get into the polling station, what chance do we have of being able to stand for office? Until these problems are resolved, there will never be enough local councillors with disabilities to represent the population. And certainly not enough disabled Members of Parliament.

Disabled Facilities – Open to All

Here in the UK, the Disability Discrimination Act of 1995 (the DDA) was a major step forward in disability rights in the UK. It's constantly being amended and expanded, although there are some significant omissions, too. I quote the Government's own website in saying that, "Service providers have to make 'reasonable adjustments' to the way they deliver their services so that disabled people can use them."

Of course, the actual definition of that word *reasonable* will keep lawyers in business for many years to come.

In reality, a business such as a restaurant is obliged to accommodate disabled customers. This doesn't mean they have to provide a Braille menu just in case a blind person comes in – having a member of staff prepared to read it to the diner is a fair compromise. Unfortunately, accessible loos are not so easily substituted.

The DDA came into force on 1st October, 2004. I took a day's leave to conduct an unscientific survey of restaurants in Bristol, where I lived at the time. This was in connection with the charity Scope, who called it the "Free 2 Pee" campaign, with a wonderful logo based on the usual wheelchair symbol – but the person in the chair has their legs crossed...

I tried to visit ten random venues. Four of them were completely inaccessible, having steps up to the door. One manager came out to say I could be carried up the steps – but not who should do the carrying or how! Two more were quite open about not having a disabled toilet. At one venue, the staff had to open a delivery door for me; one fast food outlet appeared to have great facilities, but the cleaning gear was stored in the disabled loo and I could not get in. One venue lent me a member of staff to stand outside the door because there was no lock. Only one venue – the Walkabout Inn – had a proper, full-facility, accessible loo. Sorry, *Disabled Dunny*. I contacted the restaurants with my comments – most of them didn't respond, but one of the inaccessible ones sent me vouchers for free coffees. If only I could get in there to spend them!

Of course, once you've located an accessible toilet, there's always the possibility you've got to wait while someone else uses the facilities. Please note: I do not assume that this person is disabled, because they often aren't. Here are some excuses I've heard from able-bodied people who've used the disabled facilities and felt the need to justify themselves, followed by the answers I thought but didn't say:

"I didn't want to use the Gents 'cos I knew I was gonna leave it smelly. I wouldn't go in there if I was you."

- Thanks, mate. Where else am I meant to go?

"I'm pregnant – that's the same as a disability."

- I wish I only had to live with your problems.

"There aren't any disabled people in this office."

- So where *have* I been working for the last few years?

"I needed room to change into this dress and do my make-up."

- Now I know why you've been keeping me waiting for fifteen minutes!

"Anyone's allowed to use a disabled loo – otherwise it'd be discrimination."

- Only if all loos are made accessible.

"I've got a key for me Mum. She died last year, but the key comes in handy."

- Glad to hear someone in your family got proper use from it.

"I've got a child, I'm allowed to use any toilet I like."

- You see your child as a disability? Poor thing.

Like many disabled people, I sometimes need a toilet in a hurry and I've learnt to approach the staff in a shop or wherever I am for help. I obtained a card from the MS Society many years ago. It says *"Please help me. Because of an illness which is not infectious I need to go to the toilet urgently. Thank you"* – in four European languages! Very handy, even in the UK, as it demonstrates that I have a good reason to ask.

Things are improving and restaurants belonging to the big chains are the most likely to have proper facilities, even if they're abused. It's a good idea to have some tissues in your pocket –disabled toilets are often not well-stocked. Users need to be prepared to ask staff to remove mops and *Danger – Wet Floor* signs, but at least the facilities exist. Many pubs and restaurants keep their disabled loo locked, to prevent able-bodied punters using them. Ask a staff member (or behind the bar) for a key, which is probably a RADAR one. RADAR keys are used for a national network of locked public toilets and are available from many stockists of specialist disability products and www.radar.org.uk Be wary of buying them from unofficial sources – these are often illegal copies and likely to break or be too short to fit in the locks! RADAR are a charity: support them – not profiteers! RADAR toilets crop up in the strangest of places, from pubs to car parks; from beauty spots to youth hostels. It's a great system and I wish they'd extend it to RADAR locks on footpath gates, etc. I've bought two keys to date – I lent the first one to a family member who "forgot" to return it and I had to buy another.

At the time of writing, the majority of independent eateries still don't have wheelchair accessible toilets. Of course, help from willing members of staff can make a huge difference, but I'd love to think I could just roll into a pub and assume they had a loo I could use. Until that day arrives, I'll continue to phone ahead and check with venues. And politely turn down any invitations to pub crawls...

Does She Take Sugar?

Some people will already be grinning at the title of this chapter; it's well-known in the disabled world as shorthand for a common problem. For those who haven't come across it before, here's a quick explanation:

A wheelchair user approaches the counter in a café, her companion walking behind. On reaching the counter, the disabled person requests a coffee; but the server asks the companion, "Does she take sugar?"

This even happens when I'm on my own and the person behind me is a stranger.

The assumption is that as soon as my backside hits the wheelchair cushion, my brains leak out and I am no longer able to answer the simplest question. Despite the fact that I just ordered the coffee!

My husband – the person most likely to be with me– will ignore such questions and leave me to talk to the ignorant person who evidently doesn't want to converse with a wheelchair user. In the event of it being a stranger behind me, they're naturally embarrassed and I don't hesitate to point this out to the server. I have been known to ask to see the manager. Is this an example of people being too embarrassed to even speak to a disabled person? Or is it something deeper? Has the server made a judgement that anyone in a wheelchair is by definition incompetent? I'm not sure - but I find such behaviour inexcusable, regardless of the motive.

A server once told me she was just trying to be helpful, but I don't see how it helps to talk over my head (literally!) rather than directly to me. All I'm asking for is the courtesy of being treated like any other customer. Naturally, I'm grateful when someone offers to bring my drink to the table, but I don't expect them to do so. (I have a cup holder fixed to my wheelchair, so I can manage.)

Even when a person in a wheelchair is, for some reason, unable to answer for themselves, wouldn't it be polite to address the question directly to them until advised differently? If it's somehow "appropriate" to always address questions to the helper, rather than the person with the disability - should the question "Does she take sugar?" be addressed to a blind person's guide dog?

Kids' Ride!

Warning: This is one of those chapters with icky details. Nothing too serious, but you have been warned.

A purple off-road mobility scooter is hard to ignore. Most people react positively, from tots in pushchairs who point and gape; to teenagers telling me I'm cool or wicked; to pensioners who ask me if they can borrow it!

Occasionally, they react a little too positively.

I'd parked outside the chemist's and gone in on crutches to collect my prescriptions. When I came out, I first noticed the pushchair parked alongside, blocking the pavement whilst a woman fiddled with my scooter. Then I noticed the toddler sitting on my seat.

"Excuse me," I said.

"Do you know how to make it go?" she asked.

"It won't go anywhere without the keys. Do you mind removing your child?"

"He just wants to have a ride. Where do I get the key?"

She continued to mess with the controls while the child laughed and grabbed at everything he could reach. I decided she thought my scooter was a child's ride at the same time as spotting that the child was sitting in a puddle *on my seat*.

"Erm, it's not a toy, you know. Can you lift your child off, please?"

She glared at me. "I know what it is, it's just like his Granddad's. Have *you* got the key?"

I took a deep breath.

"Well, I'm glad his Granddad lets him ride, but I have no intention of giving my keys to a stranger. Will you please remove your child, or shall I?"

51

"Don't you touch my baby!" She grabbed the child, who started wailing at the rough handling.

I pointed at my seat cover. "Does his Granddad let him pee on it, too?"

"That's 'cos you scared him – and you shouldn't use rude words in front of a baby."

I noticed two uniformed police officers across the road and waved. They started walking over.

"You spastics are all the same. You think you own everything," she shouted, grabbing the pushchair and running down the hill.

By the time I'd explained to the police officers, she was out of sight. My explanation included a comment that she objected to my using the word "pee", but thought "spastic" was a suitable term to teach her son.

I tried to buy some wet wipes in the chemist's, thinking I could clean my seat properly when I got home – after changing into clean jeans! The staff had heard some of the conversation and insisted on bringing their own cleaning kit outside and washing the seat down for me.

Another day, I was chatting with some friends in town. One of the ladies suddenly jumped up and dashed outside. She was only gone for a moment and when she came back, she explained,

"I saw some teenage girls round your buggy. But they're only taking photos."

"Of my buggy?" I asked.

"Of themselves riding it."

By the time I got outside, they were running away, yelling abuse. The controls had all been flicked into random positions and the shopping bag on the back had been unzipped. I didn't find the chewing gum until I set off for home. It took me ages to get it off the handlebar grip and I had to throw my glove away when I couldn't get that clean.

Am I missing something? When did it become acceptable to vandalise someone else's property and call them abusive names? I know these are rare incidents, but it still happens far too frequently! When you see a parent assuming everything is available for her child's entertainment, is it really surprising that some teenagers don't know any better?

What Social Life?

Warning: Minor icky words – no details, though.

Becoming disabled tells you exactly who your friends are. I wouldn't recommend it, but there's no doubt it tests your friendships. My Dad used to say that a friend in need is a bl###y nuisance. He was joking, I know how far he would go to help friends. Not everyone is so helpful.

A disability will impact on the whole social group, not just the person who has it. You start to need friends to accommodate your illness. Many people are happy to amend plans and accept there are things you can no longer do. Others just stop returning your calls. You can't do anything to change them; like so much else in life, just shrug your shoulders and carry on as best you can.

My own disability impacts on my social circle in three main ways. Firstly, I may be too fatigued to do whatever I've agreed to do and consequently let friends down. Secondly, anywhere we go has to be reasonably accessible. Thirdly, I need a disabled-friendly loo. None of these seem too onerous, until you have to accommodate them. Friends usually understand when I let them down at short notice – the first few times it happens. Not everyone is patient after the third time! People get used to checking for ramps into pubs and restaurants and have even approached the owners on my behalf. But sometimes they're too embarrassing to check for accessible facilities. If I know where we're going, I phone ahead and ask before we go.

There have been occasions where people, for whatever reason, ignore the reality of my disability and don't even tell me they've done so.

I was in a writing group who were arranging a Christmas meal out. Several restaurants had been suggested and we voted for our favourites. I'd explained from the start that I needed an accessible toilet and was thrilled to think there were so many disability-friendly restaurants that I hadn't discovered. As we all left the meeting, someone said,

"That restaurant doesn't have a handicapped loo, does it?"

"Sorry?" I asked.

"The one we've chosen doesn't have a loo for wheelchairs. I'm sure they don't 'cos I asked for my Mum."

I froze. "Are you saying these restaurants aren't accessible? I thought people were taking that into account."

"Well, we've never had the problem before. You can't expect everyone to make a special effort when the restaurants don't."

"So I can't come on the meal," I replied.

"Don't be silly, of course you can come. But you don't know how difficult it is to find a restaurant that provides for disabled people," she said.

The group discussion continued by email, with me repeating that I needed proper, accessible facilities and other people telling me I couldn't insist on that because I would be forcing them to go somewhere that had a disabled toilet. I suggested we went to the restaurant that came second in the vote – our local Italian, which has proper facilities.

Another member of the group approached me.

"You'll be on crutches for the meal, so you can manage in a normal loo. You're just trying to make us go to your favourite restaurant," she said, not meeting my eyes.

55

"I can't guarantee I won't need my wheelchair," I replied. "And even on crutches, I can't cope in a normal loo."

"So how do you manage at our meetings?"

"I don't even know where the loos are in that building. But a meeting is one thing – going out for a large meal and a long evening is another matter," I explained, already uncomfortable at being made to defend myself.

"But *why* do you have to have special treatment?"

Well, I don't think it's any of her business, but I did my best to tell her that I needed the extra space of a disabled cubicle, a sink close by and level access, without going into any specifics about my requirements. She excused herself and hurried away, looking understandably embarrassed.

A few days later, I got a phone call from yet another member of the group.

"I've got a solution to your problem," she said.

"Sorry?" I'm not very witty when something comes out of the blue like that.

"I'll buy you a packet of baby wipes. Out of my own pocket."

"Erm, why?" Like I said, not my most sparkling conversation.

"So you can use the normal facilities," she explained.

The penny dropped.

"That conversation was meant to be private! What makes you think baby wipes are all I need?"

"That's what you told ####. You just need to wash your hands."

I took a deep breath.

"That isn't what I said. Don't you think I would buy them myself, if that's all it took?"

So I left the group. They felt that it wasn't necessary for them to accommodate my disability, because it was inconvenient for them to do so; that it was appropriate to insist I defend my need for "special treatment" – but blame me for embarrassing them; to make assumptions about my disability but accuse me of using it to get my own way.

Not to mention thinking that the problems associated with a disability can be resolved with a few baby wipes.

Disability Hate Crime

"My husband would cross the street to avoid a handicapped person," she said. I'd known her for years and never expected to hear such a statement.

"So he'd avoid me, for example?" I asked.

"Well, yes. But only because he doesn't know you," she replied.

"Why?"

"It's just his way. He's always done it."

"But what's he got against disabled people?"

"No, you've got it wrong. He doesn't dislike them. He just prefers not to have them near him."

Hmm. I thought our society had grown out of thinking we should lock people away in asylums or "special homes". Apparently these Victorian ethics are alive and thriving here in the 21st Century.

It's long been known that giving bad behaviour a name makes it easier to report, but somehow more acceptable, too. In the past it happened for been road rage and binge drinking, now we have disability hate crime. The term is even mentioned in a leaflet distributed by our local police force. It's good to see they're taking it seriously, but I can't help wondering if they're also legitimising it.

The sort of behaviour I'm talking about ranges from name-calling to arson attacks. Recent media coverage has highlighted extreme cases, including some where people have died. Attacks of all kinds usually focus on the visibly disabled, especially those in wheelchairs or with severe mental health difficulties. It's hard to get accurate statistics, but it appears that serious victimisation is rare and long may this continue. The media are less interested in the low-level incidents we face every day of the week.

How low do these crimes go? Well, I've seen people cross the street to avoid me when I'm in my wheelchair - and not just when the pavement is narrow, either. Of course, it's possible that they have an irrational fear of people wearing purple or with waist-length hair – but I think my disability is the most likely cause of their discomfort. Shop assistants suddenly realise they have to be elsewhere just as I ask them for assistance; bar staff get an urge to rearrange their display of spirit bottles.

Talking to other disabled people, I hear about dog owners who encourage their dogs to foul a front garden and leave it there for the disabled resident. Name-calling is a common problem and not being served in shops, etc. At a recent disability event, I couldn't get near to a stall to buy a bottle of water, as a woman was blocking the front of the stall with her kids' bikes. Several other people were served before I could get near enough.

Although it's important that we deal with the serious crimes that are perpetrated under this heading, there's also a need to acknowledge the minor nastiness that goes on all the time. These may not be crimes – they may not even be due to actual hatred of disabled people; but are they truly acceptable in a civilised society? I am no more likely to have something contagious than the next person. Apart from my MonSter, I'm a very healthy person. But people feel they're justified in treating me as some sort of pariah. I wonder if they'd prefer we established some kind of wheelchair-accessible leper colony and migrated the disabled population to it? I am joking, by the way – not offering to move there to save other people from the offensive sight of my purple wheelchair.

Begging on the Street

I'm often invited to take part in events specifically as a disabled person. At worst, this means being the "token" wheelchair user when the organisers want to be seen to include people from all parts of society. At best, it means that the organisers do want to involve everyone and hope that my participation will encourage others to join in.

This chapter is not about the best such event I've ever been to.

What follows is taken from an email I sent to the co-ordinators after the event. They forwarded my comments to the organisers, but I did not receive a satisfactory answer and have not asked permission to quote their words here. I have edited out all names and places, as this isn't about pointing the finger; it's about demonstrating the poor treatment disabled people still receive in 21st Century Britain. I've changed the name of the organisers to "The Council" and the group who asked me to attend to "Disability Co-Ordination". The location of The Museum is similarly removed.

To: Disability Co-ordination

Dear Ladies,

I would like to thank you for inviting me to attend the day of events organised by The Council on Saturday, at The Museum. I appreciate that you were not the organisers of the day, and I would like to state that my following comments are in no way to be interpreted as a complaint about anyone at Disability Co-Ordination.

I am aware that you were invited to bring a few of your members as representatives of the disabled community who have achieved something in an artistic field. However, I feel that were all misled as to our role on the day. We were under the impression that we were being given an opportunity to talk to members of the public who were attending the events, and to sell our various products (books in my case). I accepted your invitation for two reasons: firstly, I am grateful to Disability Co-Ordination for events that have been organised in the past, and therefore like to support you; secondly, I thought it would be a pleasant day, spent chatting with people who are interested in the arts and selling sufficient books to make it worthwhile.

So what went wrong?

There were a number of items on the Programme for Day Event that were not evident on the day. Several of the arranged exhibitors did not attend. I cannot help but wonder if they realised how poorly the event was being organised?

As far as I am aware, there was no advance publicity for the event. When we made enquiries, we were informed that a "large amount" of money had been spent on advertising, including adverts on the local commercial radio station and the local newspaper. I listen to that radio station a lot, and I have heard no mention of this event at all. One lady who spoke to me on the day commented that she would have come prepared to buy items if she'd known about it. When I mentioned the advertising, she informed me that she reads the local newspaper every night ("cover to cover") and had seen nothing about any such event. Finally, I noticed that the day was not even mentioned in the Museum's own leaflet for November to February. Whatever money was spent on publicity, it was wasted.

It became clear in the course of the day that the few people who passed our stalls were either visiting the museum or the coffee shop. They did not expect to find a number of disabled artists there. I have never spent a day in such an embarrassing situation. Several people who walked past were "blanking" us – I noticed a few actually holding a hand at the side of their face, and watched one who held his mobile phone against his ear, without it ringing or his pressing a button. Disabled people are often accused of being paranoid about such behaviour, but I do not believe anyone could deny the level of wilful unawareness that was displayed on that day. Even the people who represented the organisers avoided our stalls. I have never attended an event as an "invited" exhibitor where even the organisers don't buy a single book. The film crew who were recording the event did not speak to us. The only occasion I noticed them pointing their camera at me was when I was eating my lunch, and I would have appeared in the background of something else they were filming. I did not know until the day that there was a separate evening event, to which we were not invited. Events like this only work if you either invite people to attend, or site them at a venue where a significant amount of passing foot traffic can be expected. The Museum had very few visitors on that Saturday, and they were not inclined to inspect our stalls, let alone purchase our products.

  To summarise, I feel that we (and our respective helpers) were asked to attend purely to tick the box of disabled involvement. The performers were paid for their work, I'm sure the celebrity who presented the evening event was paid for her involvement, but Disability Co-Ordination were expected to give their time for free, and endure the embarrassment of unsympathetic strangers.

  I do appreciate that you informed us we can claim travelling expenses (and I will do so in a follow-up email), but I think that we should have been given more to attend. The performers were paid to be there, the Henna Tattooists were paid, and I'm sure the organisers were not doing this work on their own time. So why were Disability Co-Ordination representatives left out? It occurred to me after the event that we were filling a traditional role for disabled people. We were attempting to engage unsuspecting passers-by in conversation with the intention of getting them to buy something from us. I've heard of this sort of occupation before – we were begging. Disability Co-Ordination were begging. No wonder they put us on the part of The Museum known as "The Street".

As ever, many thanks to all of you at Disability Co-Ordination for your sterling work.

Yours sincerely,

Meg Kingston
Writer

What do I Miss Now I'm Disabled?
Never complain about growing old – it's a privilege denied to many.

I'm surprised how often I'm asked what I miss from my pre-disability days, - and I often return the surprise by insisting there are positive aspects to my disability.

Yes, I miss the obvious things. I've never owned a bicycle in my life –I was the only kid in our village who didn't have a bike, so my feet were my only real transport. I used to walk for miles, sometimes with a rucksack of camping gear on my back. I enjoyed the mindless exercise of running and for the first few years of disability I dreamt about it. I don't any more – I think my body has forgotten what it feels like.

My worst symptoms is fatigue and it's very difficult to explain MS fatigue to anyone who hasn't experienced it. It's different to "normal" tiredness and it can happen with no warning and for no good reason. Getting more sleep won't cure it and brief physical exercise usually doesn't make it any worse. I can minimise the risks of it incapacitating me by taking things easy for a few days before an event, but it's no guarantee. *What I really miss is being able to assume I'll be alright on the day.*

Happiness is having a body that does what it's meant to.

In recent years, my MonSter has stopped me wearing contact lenses, so I'm back to glasses and miss being able to open the oven door without everything misting up. One of my great delights in wearing contact lenses was being able to walk in the rain and see where I was going. No chance of that now!

I have to plan everything nowadays. Attending a wedding at the other end of the country feels like I'm organising an invasion. Sometimes I think my whole life revolves around ramps and disabled toilets. Can you imagine being stuck on a train without a loo for three hours? I don't have to imagine!

It's very hard to be spontaneous when you need to ring ahead to ask each pub if they have steps at the entrance or narrow doorways. I remember when I only needed to check my diary before accepting an invitation, instead of phoning the venue and playing an embarrassing game of "Twenty Questions" to ensure I would be able to get in.

Holidays are particularly difficult to organise. Not only do I need to be fairly sure of ramps in the right places and wide doorways, but the weather has a direct impact on the degree of my symptoms. Unseasonable heat or humidity can leave me unable to visit the attractions or see the sights as I'd planned. Yes, I can struggle to a certain extent, but there are limits to my ability to compensate for our changing climate. Since we've known about the progressive nature of my condition, we've made an effort to do certain things whilst I'm still able. There were trips I would like to have made but never will because we didn't know my disablement would be permanent until the damage was severe enough to stop me going. But I've been luckier than many people in that regard.

I appreciate that many of these aspects apply to everyone as they age, but a disability brings them on much earlier and the unpredictable nature of MS adds a lot of unpredictability to any plans.

I miss being able to blend into a crowd, to be just another person. Nowadays, the first thing most people notice about me is the wheelchair. First impressions count, and in my case – that's the disability. They may notice my green eyes, long hair or personality – but only *after* spotting my wheels. I prefer to stand out because of my achievements, rather than the fact of my MS.

There *are* positive aspects to my disability, too. The obvious one is my writing career. I only started writing after I'd retired on health grounds and you would not be reading this book if I were still working in an office for fifty hours a week.

Although I know my long-term prognosis is bad, I refuse to let it cripple me with fear. I don't dwell on the missed opportunities in my past or worry about the future, although I acknowledge them both. Living with a chronic, progressive illness has given me a different perspective on everything in my life. I see no point in worrying about details or bearing grudges. Life is too short to waste and far too precarious to take for granted.

Carpe diem! Seize the day, for tomorrow may be too late.

And the silly thing I miss most? Dancing when no-one's watching.

Orange Juice

You Shouldn't Eat That

Warning: This is one of those chapters with icky details. Nothing gory, but I mention toilet problems in passing.

The UK population seems obsessed with diet. Whether you judge by the number of fad diets that appear every January, or the frequent Government guidelines on diet, weight and waistlines, it's a hard conclusion to dismiss. I believe most people have a fairly good grasp of what healthy eating means, but probably not how they should apply those principles to themselves; especially if they need to take a disability into account.

I've lost count of the number of people who've told me there are certain foods I either must eat, or avoid completely. The advice is rarely backed by evidence, often contradictory, and I usually only listen to the first few sentences and then make non-committal noises until I can change the subject.

Most rules for healthy eating apply to disabled people as for the rest of the population. There's no denying that lots of fresh fruit and vegetables are good for us, too much sugar is definitely not, alcohol consumption should be kept to a sensible level and short-term diets rarely work. But there are also specific points that should be considered.

Firstly, anyone who isn't very mobile will have problems with their digestive system. It's inevitable. As well as symptoms caused directly by a disability, the human body works best when it's active. If you don't walk much, you *will* suffer from constipation - and don't I wish someone had warned me about that one! Not to mention that you're likely to burn up fewer calories. Foods rich in fibre are vital, so low-carbohydrate diets are probably not a good idea. Learn to love your greengrocer – you'll be seeing a lot of her in the future.

Many people with limited mobility drink very little water so they don't have to dash to the toilet too often. This may be a mistake, as reducing fluid intake exacerbates or even causes all kinds of bladder problems, especially urinary infections. Despite the difficulties, it's very important to drink enough.

One big difference between healthy eating for most people and the same for people with MS, is over our old friend *fat*. Many people try to reduce the amount of fat in their diet, practically cutting it out if they're trying to lose weight. But MSers have to be aware that myelin is made of fat. Yes, that insulation round the spinal cord is a fatty tissue. So cutting fat out of your diet could have a negative impact on your MS symptoms.

So that's my simple dietary advice for MSers: lots of fibre and don't cut out the fat completely. But the advice from other sources can be far more drastic. Inevitably, any condition as unpredictable as MS has people who make claims of a "miracle cure". A lot of these claims centre around diet and some MSers become serial experimenters, following one set of rules for a while, then moving on to a different diet. It's possible that one of these regimes did result in a drastic improvement in one person's symptoms – but that could just as easily be due to a remission. The only way to tell for certain would be a large-scale trial, and that isn't likely to happen as there's little profit in giving dietary advice.

I'm not saying dietary changes won't improve symptoms, but I remain very cynical about them. I've tried a few in my time, but experienced no significant improvement.

Here are just a few examples of restrictions I've come across:

- Cut out cow's milk products, replace with sheep's milk products only.
- Cut out cow's milk products, replace with goat's milk products only (and don't try suggesting these two are the same, apparently they're completely different!).
- Cut out all milk products of any description (make sure you take a calcium supplement).
- Cut out chocolate, cheese, red meat, alcohol, caffeine and anything else you enjoy. Misery is good for us.
- Cut out all citrus fruits and anything derived from them.
- Go vegetarian (to various points on the scale of what's allowed and what isn't).
- Eat a few cloves of raw garlic with every meal. (It may work – but you'd have no friends left!)
- Eat a gluten-free diet. This is getting easier with more products readily available, if you want to try it.
- Avoid all processed or refined food, including anything made with white flour, refined sugar, etc.
- Avoid anything that wouldn't grow naturally in your own area. Apparently imports are the problem.

I have not included the more extreme regimes I've come across. I'm not convinced that drinking several litres of a proprietary brand of cola every day is good for anything but that company's profits. I think a lot of ideas are based on the principle "If a little is good, more is better". Personally, I think moderation is a better approach.

Another common diet problem with MS seems to be that MSers develop food allergies, or their existing ones become more acute. I'm not aware of this being officially recognised, but I've heard it anecdotally from several people. Just another little complication to make sure life with the MonSter never gets boring!

Every now and then, someone will tell me they've read an article / heard about something on the news / saw something on the internet and they have the cure for MS (and lots of other chronic conditions, I'm sure). All you have to do is follow their dietary advice. It can be hard to explain that you did try a dairy-free diet for six months and reverted when it didn't do any good. It's even harder to tell them that you're not going on the Atkins lo-carb diet, no matter how good they think it is. I've heard the case for a vegan diet several times but decided not to follow it.

On holiday a few years ago, I had trouble with one of our table companions (whose wife was vegetarian). At one meal, I had the vegetarian option for a starter, as I'm allergic to prawns. He spent the rest of the holiday telling me in his limited English that I shouldn't be eating most of the things I did, as they had meat in them. No matter how much I tried to explain, he still insisted I should follow a vegetarian diet (even though he didn't himself). I never quite decided whether he genuinely thought I was vegetarian and too stupid to understand which dishes included meat; whether he thought a veggie diet would relieve my symptoms; or whether he just thought there would be more for him if I switched to the vegetarian choices. It was very strange and extremely uncomfortable.

Another contentious subject is that of food supplements. I know many disabled people take so many vitamin and mineral tablets you can hear them rattle. Once again, I apply a healthy cynicism to the whole issue. There may be benefits for anyone taking a vitamin C supplement in the cold season, and a calcium top-up for a person who doesn't get much milk is probably a good idea. (Osteoporosis is more likely and often more problematic for people with mobility problems.) There's some evidence that vitamin D deficiency can cause all sorts of problems and most people in the UK get too little sunlight to produce their own. Many MSers take oil capsules, whether plant- or fish-derived, to ensure their myelin isn't starved of fat. It's also worth knowing that MS (and other conditions that affect the bowels) often reduce the body's ability to extract vitamin B12 from the diet, which can result in pernicious anaemia. The whole subject is a matter of personal choice and people can make up their own minds about what might help them. But one very important word of advice – beware of suggestions from people who just happen to make a profit from the product they're advocating. If someone tells you that the beneficial characteristics of a particular oil only occur if it's been prepared in a certain way and they just happen to know of the only supplier, be sure to sprinkle their words with a large pinch of salt before swallowing them. There are even books published which appear to be marketing a product in this way; a quick internet search may reveal the author's connection with the company or the patented refining process. It's possible that one of these products may be the miracle cure we're all hoping for, but if you find yourself reaching for your credit card, make sure you do so with your eyes open. Alternatively, contact me via the website and I'll sell you this bottle of snake oil for a special, unrepeatable price.

Whilst it seems unlikely that dietary changes alone are going to cure MS, there's no doubt that poor diet can exacerbate symptoms of any chronic illness. Just remember that any adjustments in your diet are more likely to be beneficial if they're long-term. A healthy diet is for life, not just for relapses.

Save me from Good Intentions!

On learning that someone has a disability, some people react positively and help as best they can. Many think they're helping, but actually make things worse. A certain type of person likes to be *seen* to help more than they actually want to do any good.

A recent conversation in a local coffee shop:

"So how's Meg?" asked the woman behind the counter.

"Ticking over, you know," I replied.

"Are your legs hurting?"

"Don't ask," I said, shaking my head.

"Ok, I won't. Is it very bad?"

"Please don't ask."

"It must be terrible for you. You know I'm here if you ever want to talk to someone. Do your legs hurt a lot of the time?"

I walked away. I know it's rude of me, but it's the politest way I could think of to end the conversation. She waited until I was settled with my coffee and sat down opposite.

"Do you often get days when it hurts this much?"

I sigh. "I said *don't ask* – what did you think I meant?"

"Oh, I know just what it's like to be noble about your suffering. Why's it suddenly hurting you so much?"

"DON'T ASK!" This time I said it loud enough for everyone to hear, before getting up, leaving coins with my unfinished coffee, and exiting.

Now, I don't know whether she genuinely thinks she's helping me or is just trying to make herself look good by listening to the poor handicapped person's problems. What I do know is that I don't appreciate someone bullying me into talking about something I don't want to discuss. The worst part is that people are most likely to behave this way when I'm least able to cope with it politely, so I'm only too likely to offend. Maybe I should have told her it wasn't pain but muscles spasms that were bothering me, and that they weren't in my legs; but I don't see what business it is of hers.

Eating Out

"Do you have a disabled toilet?" I asked the portly Duty Manager who'd refused to give me his name.

"Listen, luv. When the monks built this place in the eleventh century, they didn't worry about things like wheelchair access," he replied. "And we're a listed building so it's no good trying to sue us."

I didn't bother to point out that even listed buildings are legally obliged to comply with the Disability Discrimination Act by making "reasonable adjustments"; especially when only part of their building is listed and they completely refurbished their restaurant recently. I find the biggest obstacle is often the people who are meant to provide a service, but you can't spend your entire life prosecuting businesses that don't want your custom.

Same question, different venue – a local pub, also a listed building.

"Have you got a disabled loo?"

"We can't change the building, so I'm afraid we haven't got a proper accessible toilet. But I've fixed a grab bar in the ladies," explained Nick, the pub's co-owner. "And if you like, we can station someone outside, so you can have the whole room to yourself."

See the difference? People's attitude can be the biggest aid to accessibility, too. The landlord and staff at this pub will do anything they can to assist their less-able customers. They don't patronise us, they don't make a fuss; they're just happy to carry someone's drink to their table or help in any way. The *listing* that won't allow them to widen doorways also forbids changes to the building's facade, but if I knock on the window they'll open the side gate so I can get round the back for level access. They've asked me to tell them if I can think of anything else that would help. It's not perfect – but they make the effort and that's what it takes to make a customer feel welcome.

Guess which venue sees my money in their till?

Most places fall somewhere between these two extremes. I've been to:

- The restaurant whose function room is reachable on wheels – but only through the tradesman's entrance, kitchen and goods lift.
- A theatre where the so-called accessible loo is a stall in the ladies' and is too small even for my little manual wheelchair.
- The pub where the staff told me the accessible toilet is "only for pensioners and people with handicapped children".
- Our local Italian restaurant where the manager automatically reserves us the table in the corner, so my crutches can be propped up safely out of the way.
- The coffee shop whose response to my complaint about their high doorstep was to send me vouchers for free coffees I can't get in to buy!
- A restaurant manager who suggested I should "go before I left home" rather than expecting him to provide an accessible toilet.
- A conveyor-belt sushi restaurant where the waiter holds the stool steady so I can scramble onto it, then places my wheelchair where I can see it until I'm ready to leave.
- The pub where the doormen had to ask the manager if I was allowed to bring my crutches inside as they're meant to confiscate anything that could be used as a weapon!
- The restaurant manager who said I could use the facilities in their only accessible hotel room – unless someone was booked in it that night!

- A coffee shop where they want to move my crutches "safely out of the way" whilst I'm sitting at a table.
- The pasta restaurant whose staff fetch their movable ramp if they see a wheelchair approaching.

In most of these, the real difference lies in the attitude of the staff. Someone who ensures my wheelchair is visible to me and keeps an eye open for me waving is a help. Someone trying to take my crutches away without even telling me where they're going to put them is not a help. For that matter, I don't understand why my crutches are a trip hazard when bags of shopping aren't.

The DDA is fairly recent legislation and there's a lot of confusion about how accessible restaurants and entertainment venues have to make their premises, largely due to the vague wording of the Act itself. (What *is* a "reasonable adjustment"?) There isn't anyone to report infringements to; our only recourse is to sue. As long as some companies prefer making excuses to addressing the issue, this vagueness will cause arguments and make lawyers a lot of money. I haven't taken anyone to court over access yet and if I ever do, an MS charity will get a cheque from me. It's not about the money – it's about equality.

Some businesses are willing to make the effort whilst others wait until they're threatened with legal action. I'm informed that the restaurant mentioned at the start of this chapter now has accessible facilities, but they still don't have me as a customer. As well as sending letters of complaint, I will continue to speak with my wallet and support those who value my custom.

Spending Pounds to Spend Pennies

It strikes me as beautifully ironic that it costs thousands of pounds to build and equip a toilet that enables a wheelchair user to *spend a penny*. Ironic, but painfully true – and probably the reason so few truly accessible toilets exist.

A while ago, the writing group I belonged to were arranging a Christmas meal. We'd pick a restaurant and book a large table for ourselves and our significant others. I was looking forward to it and was thrilled to see how many venues were suggested – I didn't realise there were so many nearby that offered disabled facilities. Then someone dropped the bombshell – our chosen restaurant didn't have a disabled toilet. I pointed out that I wouldn't be able to go, and had made them aware of this from the outset I needed these facilities.

"Well – you don't realise how difficult it is to find anywhere that has a disabled toilet."

- Actually, I have a pretty good idea. Welcome to my world.

"That's not our problem."

- No, it's not. Thanks for thinking of me.

"You should complain to the restaurant, not us."

- I could, but I don't think they'll build an accessible toilet before Christmas.

"You go to places that don't have handicapped toilets all the time."

- Not for a meal, I don't.

"Other people have special needs, too. You just assume you're the only one."

- I'm happy to take other people's needs into account – but I was the only one who mentioned anything.

79

"I'll buy you some baby wipes so you can use a normal toilet."

- I'm not sure what you think my problem is – and I'm even less willing to tell you the details!

"You can't expect everywhere to have special facilities, just for you."

- Well, the law expects them to. Would you go to a restaurant that didn't allow you to use the toilet?

"Can't you just wait until you get home?"

- Would you?

Apparently my responses were offensive and I failed to take into account other people's feelings. I was removed from the email circulation list and effectively excommunicated from the group. The self-elected committee refused to answer my emails; other members of the group were told I'd gone off in a huff because they wouldn't go to my favourite restaurant – which is the only one on the list that does have proper, accessible facilities. Frankly, I'd been looking forward to finding a new eatery – but there needs to be a toilet I can use! It's nice to be wanted.

Once you start looking around, it's amazing how many public venues don't provide disabled toilets. I've heard so many excuses over the years I've thought about writing a book about them. Oh, hang on – I am doing that.

Drugs on Trial

When you're well, you have a million wishes. When you're ill, you only have one.

Many treatments are available for multiple sclerosis; both disease-modifying and symptomatic. Or to put it another way, ones that try to reduce the MS itself and ones that treat one symptom at a time.

This book is not designed to advise anyone on the best type of treatment –that's a choice to be made with qualified healthcare professionals. There are new disease-modifying drugs (DMDs) available every year and an MS nurse or neurologist will be best placed to advice on the suitability of those. Drugs are also available which can help with symptoms including: pain, fatigue, muscle spasms, etc.

To ensure that new drugs are safe to use, each one goes through a testing process for several years. There is a constant need for people to participate in these trials and I've done a few. Commercial drug trials are always double-blind – meaning that neither the volunteer nor the medical staff know whether the tablets administered contain the drug being tested or a placebo.

One trial was for a cannabis-derived drug being tested by the National Health Service. My participation involved day visits to a local hospital, where I underwent a detailed series of physical and emotional tests each time, before being given the tablets. The staff were friendly, helpful and willing to answer questions; my consultant neurologist was part of the team responsible for the trials. As it was an NHS trial, I did not receive any payment – not even my travelling expenses. I took the tablets as required, kept a log of my symptoms over the period, returned for all follow-up appointments and felt supported throughout the whole process. The trial ended about a year after my involvement and I received a polite letter informing me what I had been taking and that the drug had moved into the next stage of the ratification process.

Another trial was a big, multi-national one being run by a private company, whose UK operations were based at a London hospital. Volunteers were paid for their involvement – a lump sum, plus expenses and a payment to the person who referred them in the first place. We were subjected to a lot of very expensive tests and I was told the results of my initial testing would be sent to my GP and neurologist. (The final test results would be a secret, due to the possibility of the drug doing me some good!) The trial involved several stays in their ward – equipped with an assortment of old furniture from the host hospital. Some staff were very friendly, others treated us poorly. One administrator phoned me on the Thursday before my planned admission on the Saturday, to say that I had to come on Friday morning instead. She had phoned my driver to change the arrangements – before speaking to me! I insisted that I couldn't re-plan my life at such short notice and travelled in as planned on the Saturday. I was not the only volunteer to feel that this administrator thought they owned us for the duration of the trial.

The trial has now ended – I received an oddly-phrased letter when the results demonstrated that the new drug was no better than placebo treatment. I never received my full expenses and the person who referred me did not get anything, either – despite numerous emails and phone calls to the company. I have not been informed whether I was on the drug itself or a placebo. The promised letters were never sent to my GP and neurologist. The same administrator has since been in touch to tell me I need to come back for another assessment. I insisted I was not travelling without a written guarantee that they would cover all my expenses. She did not call again. Other people on the same trial had similar problems with the same administrator. Some of us are still in touch, even though we've refused to give any more of our time to the company who brought us together.

So – one trial with minimal budget, who treat the volunteers with gratitude and courtesy. Another where we were paid for our involvement (if not all that was promised) and treated rudely. Take your pick.

Despite the problems, I'm glad to have made my contribution to medical advances in this way. I couldn't have done it when I was working full-time and the trial requirements exclude anyone whose disability has progressed beyond a certain level. I made good use of my window of usefulness by taking part. And I met some great people!

Anyone wishing to volunteer for a trial should speak to a medical professional. Private companies actually pay for advertisements in the national press (and Facebook!), whereas NHS trials are publicised through the medical profession and the websites of charities such as the MS Society.

Adapt and Survive

With any form of chronic illness or disability, there is a need to cope with changing circumstances. Whether it's the condition itself that is worsening, or a steady increase in disability due to inactivity, most people will be aware that they need to adapt to changes. Adapt to survive.

When Martin moved in with me, we divided the household jobs up, so that we each did the chores we were good at, a share of the ones either of us could do and a few of the ones neither of us wanted. A few years after we were married, my physical difficulties – which turned out to be MS – started to affect the types of jobs I could do. So we shuffled the list a little. And so we've continued. If I can't do something, either Hubby has to do it or we pay someone else. Some jobs get done less often than they used to. A few don't get done at all. If you think it's important for a house to be kept spotlessly clean and tidy – don't visit me. Our home is clean enough to be healthy, but definitely lived-in!

Sometimes there are ways to make a job easier – gadgets that do some of the work, or buying prepared food instead of making everything from scratch. So if I serve pastry, it's a safe bet that I bought it ready-made. And the veg for my home-made soup was probably chopped up in the food processor. Making one job easier leaves me with the energy to do something else.

For obvious reasons, it's harder for me to get up and go into another room when I need something, so I tend to have duplicates which are close at hand when I need them. There are pens, notepads and scissors in just about every room; I have at least two books being read; there's one half-knitted item in the lounge, another in the bedroom – and so on.

A friend once commented, politely, on the amount of clutter around my seat in our lounge.

"It's so I don't have to fetch anything when I need it," I explained.

"But you *can* go get things, so why not wait until you want it?" asked Ian.

"Because it's tiring, so I try to reduce the number of times I have to get up."

"It can't be that tiring just to go get a pair of scissors," he was trying to see my problem.

"Not if it's just once. But how many times do you get up and down in an evening?" I asked.

"A few times. Five or six, maybe."

"I bet it's more than that," I said. "Can I suggest something?"

"Erm, you want me to count how often I stand up each evening?"

"No – I was going to suggest another way for you to realise how often you get up."

"I'm not sure I'm going to like this," he replied, grinning.

"I suggest you hit your leg every time you're about to get up. You can borrow my leatherworking mallet if you want. Don't give yourself bruises, but do it hard enough to hurt," I explained.

"And that's what it feels like when you stand up?" he asked.

"No – but it'll make you aware of how often you get up," I said. "You'll soon start keeping things to hand and planning to fetch everything in one trip."

I don't think he actually did this – but he did get a better picture of why I've adapted my lifestyle around my disability.

It *is* difficult to understand if you don't have a chronic illness. I've can tell you that my day is effectively shorter because of my fatigue and I can talk about having less energy than most people, but it's doesn't mean much if you haven't experienced it. My favourite metaphor is known as the *beer-mat story*. Or spoons, sweets, or cigarettes –whatever comes to hand!

Let's say we have a pile of beer mats in front of us and I'm trying to explain this to you. I pass you a handful of mats, about a dozen or so. Then I explain that they represent my energy for the day. It's your job to decide what I'm going to do with them.

It takes about four beer-mats worth of energy just to get through the day – even if I do nothing but sit around. Two beer-mats to have a shower, one more to get dressed. Cooking dinner for the two of us will take three more, going out for a meal only takes two – but dressing smart and doing hair and make-up takes two more! By the time I've listed everything in a "normal" day, there aren't many beer mats left to do anything else. An hour's writing takes two mats – a couple of phone calls eat up another one. If I'm going into town (three beer-mats), something else has to get left out. That's bad enough – but at the start of the day I don't know how many beer mats I've got to play with. Sometimes I get to mid-afternoon and find I've run out. So I have fewer beer-mats than most people and I don't know how many I have until they run out.

It's that simple!

I've known disabled people who try to hoover their house every day, clean the windows every weekend and iron everything they wear. And they wonder why they don't have the energy left to do anything fun. Life is too short to iron your underwear! Well, it is for me. Of course, there are people who prefer to spend their energy on keeping their house immaculate – that's their choice. I'm just not that house-proud. So if I haven't tidied my lounge before you visit, I've probably used my beer-mats for writing or something instead.

Custard Yellow

When to Tell

Although most people's MS is classed as "relapsing-remitting", symptoms will gradually worsen over time. After each remission, the MSer recovers slightly less of their function than before. This isn't just the MS itself – a relapse saps energy, tightens muscles and generally makes it harder to do anything. The human body doesn't cope well with periods of enforced inactivity and is reluctant to recover fully. The same applies to most forms of disability and chronic illness – its impact is likely to increase.

So, having accepted that the MonSter is here to stay and resigned to the steady deterioration in mobility etc., the question is: When do you tell anyone else? Do you wait until it's obvious something's wrong – like needing a stick to walk? Do you tell them as soon as you know yourself, so they understand what you're going through, even before it affects your relationship? Do you deny that there's a problem and put everything down to clumsiness? These are not trivial questions.

Starting with your nearest and dearest. Partner or parent, spouse or significant other - they'll almost certainly know something is wrong. They'll have noticed your medical appointments, spotted you borrowing books from the library or researching on the internet. Often, they'll be relieved to hear your diagnosis, as they've been imagining the worst. You may even find they've noticed symptoms you weren't aware of, but didn't want to mention.

At some point, you'll decide to "come out" to your friends. I personally told a few close friends soon after my diagnosis, but many acquaintances didn't get to hear for quite a while. Some people announce it almost formally, others prefer to casually mention it in passing. It's a tough stage to go through and a good time for friends to cut the sufferer a little slack.

A young MSer I know agonised over when he should mention his MS (which isn't obvious) to someone he's dating. Should he be up-front and mention it on a first date? Wouldn't it be harder to explain later why he didn't mention it before? What about speed-dating? (Personally, I feel that 2 minutes isn't much time to get to know someone anyway, and I wouldn't mention a disability.)

There comes a point when your disability is common knowledge. Word gets around - people know about it without you telling them. Things can be uncomfortable for a while, not knowing who's heard, but this passes and you can relax in the knowledge that your friends won't ask why you're using a walking stick.

One of the hardest decisions is about telling your employer. On the one hand, there is an understandable fear that admitting to a chronic, progressive condition will prejudice the management against you. On the other hand, once you've admitted to a disability, it becomes possible to ask for adjustments to be made which will make your working life easier.

There is no easy solution to this dilemma. I've been completely open with my employers about my disability since my first undiagnosed symptoms and have suffered discrimination as a result. Other MSers have tried to keep it quiet, only to be criticised when the truth comes out. In theory the Disability Discrimination Act prevents negative discrimination and places the employer under a responsibility to make "reasonable adjustments" to facilitate your working for them. In practice, it often doesn't: but you can't keep MS a secret for ever.

As an openly disabled person, I have found managers very reluctant to make the accommodations I request, even when I am entitled to them by law or company policy. For example:

A manager circulated a new layout for the office. Desks were being shuffled to fit in additional people and most staff were being moved. My name appeared at the desk furthest from the door. I approached the manager and asked that I be allocated to a desk nearer the facilities.

"I can't change the plan now it's been published. You get whatever I've allocated."

"But this moves me even further from the toilet," I explained.

He cut me short. "I don't want to hear about women's problems. I've had half the Department complaining they don't want to be moved. If I make changes to suit you, they'll all expect the same."

Well, it's quite possible that they would, but that's the point where a good manager would refer to the DDA. It states that an employer has to make reasonable adjustments to accommodate disabled employees. I felt that asking to be moved to a more appropriate desk could hardly be described as an unreasonable request. In the end, I had to research the legislation which states that a disabled person's place of work should not be more than 40 yards from the nearest suitable toilet; and the Company's own policy which reduced this further to 32 yards. Only when he'd seen this in writing on a formal document would he consider implementing it. Even then, my new desk was more than 40 yards from the loo, if you measure the distance I had to travel rather than a straight line on the floor plan. He insisted it was within the 32 yards – claiming he'd walked it!

One example of an employer having better policies (on paper) than the legal restrictions, but these being ineffective because a manager wasn't prepared to follow them. HR Department's only advice was that I could bring a formal complaint against him!

I have also known managers to use the fact of my MS to their advantage and my detriment:

One manager, having heard that MS is worsened by stress, used my disability to prevent me doing anything except sit at my desk. His statements included: "You can't go on the training course, it would be too stressful for you." I've never known a training course as stressful as doing a job you haven't been trained for!

On another occasion, the team were told we'd all be going out for a meal before Christmas, as a thank-you for our work over the year. I phoned the restaurant to check about access. I was told it wasn't accessible and they weren't aware anyone in our party had special requirements. Foolishly, I approached the manager who'd announced the event. I won't quote his exact words, but the gist of it was that someone had to staff the office in case of any urgent problems, so that worked out fine for everyone. Except the person who missed out on a free meal and an afternoon off, that is!

One manager informed me that I would never be considered for promotion as the more senior roles involved a formal security check and that my disability would "obviously" prevent me from passing this. He wasn't interested in anything I had to say, just told me not to waste his time by applying.

There are many more examples I could quote, but the pattern is clear. Not only did I find it hard to get "reasonable adjustments" considered, but I also found some managers would use the fact of my disability to prevent me doing something I should have been allowed to do, or to force me to do something no-one else was expected to do. Even when the company policies are in keeping with the DDA, the reality is that it's very difficult to force a manager to be fair if they don't want to.

It's never easy to tell people about your disability, and it's likely there will be negative repercussions whether you're open about it or not. There is no simple solution and no-one can tell you when to "come out". Just remember, once you tell anyone, word will spread – you can't tell some people and keep it secret from everyone else.

Working Life

I worked for many years with my increasing disability, both before and after learning that I had multiple sclerosis. I was always as honest as possible with my employers but from the very earliest days, I experienced what I saw as discrimination. Even the smallest request that wouldn't cost anything was viewed with suspicion by the management and I usually had to produce documentation to prove that I needed or was entitled to something – even as simple as having a desk near the disabled loo instead of at the opposite end of the office. It's more relevant for me to list some of the many small examples of this behaviour, rather than a few larger ones, as it's the general atmosphere of discrimination that made office life so difficult for me. Working as a rare (sometimes the only) female in male-dominated technical teams, I experienced sex-discrimination all my working life – from being paid less than my peers to a team leader who thought a quick grope was acceptable behaviour.

But the treatment of a disabled worker by management and human resources staff takes things a lot further.

One manager seemed to assume I was faking the whole thing. He'd never actually come out and admit it, so I couldn't argue the point with him. He kept trying to prove I was only pretending, which made for a very difficult working environment. I know MS is weird, but that doesn't mean I was making it up! I offered to bring him a copy of my latest brain scan, showing the lesions caused by MS – he said it was pointless because I could easily counterfeit that!

I once tried to complain that another member of staff regularly ran through the office and even turned cartwheels down the central aisle to show off. My manager said he couldn't stop her and that it was my responsibility to keep out of her way.

Any time someone had to miss out on a perk, such as a day out, a team meal or even training courses, the person chosen to cover the office was the disabled one. When I complained that it was someone else's turn to draw the short straw, I was reminded of the importance of being a team player and that my comments would be recorded for my performance review. And they were.

At various times, I have been paid less that my peers. In one role, I was expected to interview candidates to work under me, but at a grade *higher* than my own. Once we'd appointed someone and her start date was fixed, I was offered a pay rise to a few hundred pounds a year more than she would be earning. One excuse for not re-grading me earlier was that the stress of being a higher grade would be bad for me – although I think being underpaid is far more stressful than a change in job title.

I had a grab rail fixed to the wall by my desk, which allowed me to pull myself out of my wheelchair and into my desk chair. One day it collapsed, dropping me hard onto the floor and revealing the 2" plugs holding it in place. I pointed this out to my manager, who arranged for it to be replaced – with the same plugs. It took me weeks to get it fixed in place with 6" plugs, as it should have been.

A lot of assumptions were made about what I was able to do, and decisions were made that I was expected to live with. As my "needs" had been taken into account, it was ungrateful of me to complain. I was excluded from team events (also known as "jollies") because the manager claimed they would be too tiring for me. So it was only sensible that I should stay in the office in case of any problems.

One team worked a shift system but people didn't like working night shifts on Bank Holiday weeks – we were paid an allowance for each night worked, so a Bank Holiday week meant less pay for the same amount of disruption. I was scheduled to work all but one of the Bank Holidays in the year, regardless of the usual rota.

I had great difficulty with fire evacuation procedures. In all the years that I worked in offices above the ground floor, I never left the office during a fire drill. There was an "evac-chair" in the stairwell, but the Fire Marshalls weren't prepared to use unless there was a genuine emergency. I once looked at the Fire Marshall manual, where the page about the evacuation of mobility-impaired people had only five words on it – "This Page Left Intentionally Blank". I even asked permission to try using the stairs – just to see how well I could manage if I ever needed to, but was told that doing so would breach the Company's insurance policy!

My disability was frequently used to justify my being treated differently. As MS is known to be worsened by stress, successive managers have told me they're treating me differently to avoid putting me in a stressful situation – like a training course or an interview for a better post. I was passed over for promotion because of the amount of sick leave I was assumed to have taken, even though the person appointed had taken twice the number of sick days. I was told not to apply for another promotion as the post needed a security check and it was assumed that my disability would automatically make me a security risk.

As well as the misuse of my assumed problems, there were additional pressures caused by the MS. Most staff members would go for a walk or sit in their cars for an hour's lunchbreak. As I couldn't do either, I had to eat my lunch *al desco* – at my desk. Wearing headphones, reading a book or even having a sign to say I was on my break didn't work and I often didn't even get enough time to eat my sandwiches.

I once complained to a manager that the workload was too large and that I was working fifty hours a week just to keep on top of it. He replied,
"If it takes you fifty hours to do what a normal person does in thirty, then that's what you have to do."

One of the nastier aspects of this environment is that a member of staff with a changing condition, such as my progressive MS, is expected to explain and justify any changes in their condition as they happen. So as well as suffering new or worsening symptoms, I had to explain to HR and various managers what was happening even before I understood myself. Other disabled people have told me of similar situations and of the distress this caused him, too. At the very time when you're feeling vulnerable, you have to deal with senior members of staff playing the blame game.

In the months prior to my leaving full-time work, I knew my health was worsening and made several attempts to improve my working environment. I asked permission to work more flexible hours; to work from home some of the time and even to take some unpaid leave. All of these requests were turned down. When my health eventually collapsed and I left work, it didn't take many months for me to be offered flexible working arrangements and the chance to work from home, if I'd come back into the team. Unfortunately, I have not been able to return and will probably never work full-time again, however accommodating an employer may now be.

Although the media like to make the most of the big discrimination cases, I believe it's the small things that actually make it harder for us to work with able-bodied people. It's very hard to address any of these issues without sounding incredibly petty – but they add up to an atmosphere that's very wearing. I accept that many managers don't see this as discrimination – but when only one person in a team has a disability and they are repeatedly singled out for the jobs other people don't want to do, I would say that's exactly what it is.

Difficulties in Definition

One consequence of being disabled is the need to explain your disability to the most casual of acquaintances, in a way that conveys its seriousness without any icky details. Even worse, you don't know whether the person asking has a genuine interest in your problems, or is just being casually polite. The first person may be offended by too brief an answer, the second by even the slightest detail.

The question is easier to answer when it comes from an internet friend who's never met me "in the meat world", or someone who knew me before the disability. But over the years I've been approached by complete strangers who assume they have a right to ask highly personal questions. I can be anywhere, sitting on a train or in a cafe, or just browsing in a shop, when the question comes out of nowhere. "What's wrong with you, then?" There's a real temptation to ignore the questioner, or reply just as impolitely, but I generally resist the urge.

I say "I have MS" and shrug - trying to convey that I don't want to make a big deal of it. Many people don't pursue the question, some recognise the term and know a little about the condition; but the all-too-frequent response I've learnt to dread is, "That's yuppie flu, isn't it?" So I try to explain that it's a different illness (*Why* do people assume MS and ME are the same thing?), but may still get a lecture about "Don't the doctors say that's all in your head?" It's a situation I can't win – I have a formally-diagnosed physical illness with medically defined symptoms, but people think it's a different condition that they've heard is sometimes psychosomatic. If I try to explain the difference, they're likely to be offended because they didn't want to know all the medical details! I really empathise with people who have genuine ME and have to endure the common assumption that it's not a "proper" illness, as I often find myself trying to defend its reality – as well as explaining my own illness.

Another MSer I know avoids the acronym problem by saying, "I have Multiple Sclerosis." He tells me that the misunderstanding he encounters most often is that people think he said "Multiple Cirrhosis" and assume he's an alcoholic! (Cirrhosis of the liver is often seen as self-inflicted, regardless of its many possible causes.) So that doesn't work, either.

The MS sufferers I know in the United States have a better solution. They can say, "I have MS – like Montel Williams," or Alan Osmond, as they prefer. We don't have a celebrity with MS in the UK, so that avenue isn't open to us. I could mention Jacqueline du Pre, but most people who've heard of her only remember her from the film "Hilary and Jackie" (great film, by the way) and that she "went strange and died". Not exactly a positive image! I could mention JK Rowling's late mother, but I don't think many people outside of the MS community even know that she had MS.

I believe the situation would be easier if we had an MSer in the limelight in this country, so I'll just have to hope someone with the disease achieves their 15 minutes of fame soon, giving us a parallel we can mention. (Maybe an MSer who proves to be a talented writer? Well, I can hope!)

I find it much easier with kids. Young children ask straightforward questions like "Why have you got those sticks?" "Why are you in a pushchair?" or "Why are you driving a car on the pavement?" and I can be sure they want an answer. I take enquiries from children very seriously – it's a golden opportunity to show the next generation that disabled people are still human. I make eye contact (which is particularly easy if I'm in my wheelchair) and explain that my legs don't work very well, so I use my sticks / wheelchair / buggy to get about. If they ask for more detail, I'll tell them I have an illness that affects parts of me, including my legs, but it isn't catching and it doesn't mean I'm different to other people. A lot of kids are quite jealous of my buggy and this makes it easier for them to approach me and ask when an adult wouldn't. I welcome their questions and hope I've helped in my own small way to improve the general perception of disabled people for the future.

The really odd thing about all this is that once I have explained the reason for my disability, most people have heard of MS – often because they know or have known another MSer. It's a common enough condition that there's likely to be one of us in most people's social circle.

I do empathise with those who have a less well-known condition, or one with an unsympathetic public image, such as ME or cirrhosis. I'm sure people with any medical condition suffer similar misunderstandings. I can't see a ready solution, as people can't know the details of every possible condition that can afflict others. Maybe we all need to be a little more inclined to listen attentively to what we hear about various illnesses; but simultaneously we must promise not to whinge or go into icky details. Perhaps this is a situation where we need to be a little more *childishly* honest instead of hiding behind adult concealments. In the meantime, if anyone comes up with a nice, compact way to say that they have multiple sclerosis that never causes confusion or offends anyone – then please let me know. I could really use it!

Waist-High in a Grown-up World
Warning: Contains adult humour. Nothing too explicit, but some comments may offend.

A man lives on the nineteenth floor of a block of flats. Every morning, he takes the lift to the ground floor and goes to work. When he comes home, he rides the lift to the twelfth floor on sunny days, gets out and climbs the stairs the rest of the way. On wet days, he takes the lift all the way. Why?

It's an old riddle. If you haven't come across it before, the answer is that he's a dwarf and can only reach the right button in the lift if he's carrying his umbrella.

Of course, in today's world, I should use the phrase, "person of limited stature" and probably shouldn't even tell the story. I apologise to anyone I've offended with the tale, but I think it illustrates an important point:

Being shorter than most people makes life difficult – and this is a source of humour to some.

I'm drawing a deliberate parallel between people who are significantly below average height and those of us who use a wheelchair. It's not just steps that cause problems for us.

If asked, most people would realise that being in a wheelchair makes it difficult to reach items on higher shelves in a shop. (How *do* wheelchair users buy pornography?) Some people may even realise that we can't reach lift buttons. But what else? Here are a few situations you may not have thought of:

- Bars. If you think it's hard to get served in a busy pub, you should try doing it from a wheelchair. Once you've fought your way to the front, all the bar staff can see is a disembodied hand pathetically waving money at them.
- Doors with security systems. Even if the card reader (or whatever) is in reach, you've still got to swipe your pass and pull the door open whilst moving through it. That takes four hands, if you need two to push your wheels.
- Service counters. Quite often, these are simply too high. Occasionally there's a reduced height one – but that is usually the first window closed if the bank isn't fully staffed.
- Revolving doors. There's a mechanical eye just above floor level that stops the door if anyone's too near the front or back. But there usually isn't enough room to fit a wheelchair in without tripping one or other of the sensors. I avoid revolving doors, even if it looks like it's big enough.
- Worktops. Kitchens are designed for people of average height and are too high for a wheelchair user. It's not too bad if you're just making a cuppa, but spend half an hour chopping vegetables or kneading bread and your shoulders will remind you about it all night.
- Measuring things around me. It's very difficult to judge someone's height when you're in a wheelchair. Everyone is a couple of feet taller than me – so it's hard to judge with any accuracy.

- Automatic doors. Sometimes, the sensors for these only work if you're tall enough. If I know in advance, I approach them with my arms waving. It may look stupid, but it makes the door open. If I approach one without knowing it's heightist, I hit the unopened door at speed and rebound into an embarrassed heap on the floor.

There's another problem with lifts, too. I've been known to say, "Crowded lifts smell different when you're in a wheelchair". Here comes that adult humour I warned you about...

I got into a lift with a colleague. He's a nice guy, GSOH and all that. The lift doors closed and he observed that we were alone in the lift and that he'd just noticed the height of my mouth against his own anatomy. (I'm not going to quote his actual words.) He seemed to think I should find this as funny as he evidently did. I couldn't decide whether it was more offensive to me as a woman or a disabled person, so I settled for warning him that I bite...

It's a well-documented fact that height carries advantages in many situations. In an election, the taller candidate is more likely to win. Tall people are more likely to be promoted in the workplace, served first and so on. Being in a wheelchair has the effect of reducing a person's height and therefore their status – which may account for some of the disability-related discrimination they experience, in common with people of limited stature.

Another height problem with being in a wheelchair is shopping baskets. And handbags and anything else people carry under their arms. But shopping baskets are the worst – they're hard and they have corners. I couldn't tell you the number of times I've been hit in the head by shopping baskets, or just managed to dodge them. And if I put a hand up to deflect the basket when someone's turning round, they can't understand why I'm pushing at their shopping. Isn't it obvious? Presumably not. And as for the fashion of large handbags carried under an arm – don't get me started.

Now, I'm not trying to get shopping baskets banned or stop anyone from carrying their handbag under their arm. All I'm asking for is a little thought. Just remember that it sticks out, often with hard corners, and have a moment's consideration for those of us with heads at waist height.

Gadgets

"Thanks for your help. 'Bye."

I waved as the Occupational Therapist drove away, then collapsed in a heap. He'd been sent by the Local Authority to assess my situation and see if they could offer anything that would help me. In the course of a two-hour appointment, he'd been through my home like a clipboard-wielding whirlwind. I needed to catch my breath and look through the list he'd left me with.

Most of the items the OT arranged for me to "try" went back to the distribution centre within a few weeks. Despite his good intentions, a couple of hours is obviously not enough time to assess what would actually benefit me, and he chose to give me everything he had in stock that looked even vaguely helpful for me. I was told to try them at my leisure and keep the ones that proved worthwhile. This approach worked for me, and I returned the unnecessary gadgets quickly so they could be sent out to someone who might need them more than I do. But I can't help wondering how many of these things are sat in garages and spare rooms across the country, gathering dust and getting tripped over.

Local Authorities vary more than they should across the UK. It's always worth contacting your local council and asking what they can offer.

I'm a bit of a gadget freak. I love things that do a job well and I browse catalogues and shops that sell the latest boy-toys, just to see what's out there. I don't buy many, partly because many of them are just gimmicks, but I do like to see them. So it's only natural that I pay attention to gadgets designed to make life easier for disabled people; although I'm usually disappointed in what I find.

Whether I've seen them in a catalogue, at a show like NAIDEX or courtesy of an OT, I've found the majority of gadgets don't really offer much help. I divide them into five categories – according to their highly subjective value to me.

Inappropriate: Something that just doesn't help me. In theory this shouldn't be a problem, but in practice there are so many people with an all-disabled-people-are-the-same attitude that it can become a nuisance having to explain that you just don't need this particular widget. "More expensive" does not always mean "better", neither does "new, improved" – but it's always worth a look.

Not yet: My condition is progressive – as is the case for many of us with a chronic condition. If you include age, then we all have something that will make us less able over time. In my view, it's a mistake to use an aid before you need it, but it can be difficult to explain that you'd rather keep struggling up and down stairs while you can, instead of getting that nice, shiny stair lift fitted.

Better option: Many products with a "disability" label on them are simply not as good as something else you could buy from another shop. Something designed for a person with arthritis may not help someone with reduced sensation in their hands. Not all disabilities are created equal!

Aesthetics: Things are changing, but most products aimed at helping the disabled are dull metallic, industrial grey or black. If you're going to have those crutches with you whenever you're out, don't you want them to look good, as you would with a new handbag or pair of shoes? Vanity may be a sin, but there's no reason someone with a disability should look dowdy.

Great: There are gadgets that work. I have a few that make my life a lot easier, sometimes in ways I never even thought about.

As the population ages, more companies are focussing their efforts towards less-able people. We may not be pensioners, but we are benefitting from what's known as the "grey pound". Innovations for making life easier are appearing all the time. No longer just expensive items like stairlifts, but simple products pop up and this alone is a good reason for attending exhibitions aimed at disabled people. Keep an eye open for what's out there. Even if you don't need it today, it's good to know it exists if you ever do.

Some of my favourites are gadgets I use in ways their manufacturers never intended. For example, I keep two little karabiners in my handbag. They're small versions of a clip used for climbing – about 10cm (4 inches) long, shaped like a number 8, each has two clips that fasten to straps. I use them when I'm shopping or travelling with luggage. One clip fastens to my handbag strap which is looped around my waist. The other holds the handles of bags of shopping, or whatever else I want to carry on my lap. Very simple little devices, but they make life that little bit easier.

Because my condition has gradually worsened over the years, I've found it hard to get aids through the National Health Service. I've come to realise that if you break your ankle, the NHS will provide a pair of crutches and someone will show you how to use them. (No, it's not as obvious as you might think.) If you have steadily-worsening walking difficulties, no-one ever offers them and they don't refer you to a specialist who can advise their proper use. One of the most important things for any disabled person in this position to realise is to learn to ask.

I've had several pairs of crutches in my time, all bought with my own money because I never pushed anyone into providing them. I've never been shown how to use them and had to muddle it out for myself. I am now very mobile on my crutches (when I'm able to use them) and often surprise people with how "able" I can be on four feet. But I still wish I'd asked for someone to advise me at the start. Similarly with wheelchairs. And other gadgets over the years.

Dignity, Privacy and Other Myths

The DDA is one of the few laws I know of that specifically mentions a person's right to dignity:

(1) For the purposes of section 31AA, a body subjects a disabled person to harassment where, for a reason which relates to the disabled person's disability, the body engages in unwanted conduct which has the purpose or effect of—

(a) violating the disabled person's dignity; or

(b) creating an intimidating, hostile, degrading, humiliating or offensive environment for him.

However, this is a right that is rarely respected.

I was invited to a Wedding at a venue with no lift and a "feature" staircase. Unsurprisingly, I declined the invitation. I was criticised for doing so, with the words:

"We can get some of the guys to carry you up the stairs. It'll be a laugh!"

So the guests were to manhandle me into the function room? I didn't realise I was meant to be providing the entertainment.

As with many laws, the DDA is full of such vague terminology. Lawyers get rich arguing about such details, but the person who's meant to be protected by the legislation seems to get little benefit.

I was due to have minor surgery to correct a problem caused by my MS. It wasn't serious, but it was embarrassing. I told very few people about it – always with the insistence that I didn't want it talked about. I shouldn't have bothered. My manager at work actually announced in a team meeting that I was going into hospital, but that it was only for #### and that team members would be able to phone me once I was at home, as I'd be well enough to help with their queries. So he knew better than my doctor when I would be fit to work – and he wanted to make sure everyone knew exactly what embarrassing problems I was suffering. I tackled him about this afterwards and he replied that everyone knew I was disabled, so I couldn't reasonably expect him to keep the details of my surgery secret.

In other words, a disabled person has no right to privacy in his team.

I also told one relative about the same surgery, insisting that I didn't want anyone else to know about it. The next time we spoke, she said,

"I was talking to #### about your operation,"

"What? But you told me you were going to keep it quiet," I replied.

"Yes, but her daughter's a doctor. And she might be able to help."

"And can she?"

"Of course not – it's not her area of expertise!" she said.

Correct me if I'm wrong – but I don't see any point in telling anyone about my problems if you know it's not their specialism. The same person had told the staff in the local baker's shop, too. As I found out when I went in to buy our lunch.

Another problem is the use of a disabled person as some sort of trophy. I know I've been invited to some events as the token disabled person. Some organisers want to be seen as inclusive and a person in a wheelchair is very handy for the press photos. It becomes obvious when I'm not important to the gathering, but somehow find myself positioned prominently for the local paper to take pictures.

Disabled people have as much right to privacy and dignity as everyone else – morally and legally. Yet time and again I find my medical problems are treated as something to gossip about, regardless of my wanting to keep them private. And I'm told this is acceptable because everyone can see my disability. Or my disability is used to make someone else look good, regardless of their actual behaviour.

Presenting Disabilities

Several local societies, libraries and other groups have seen the workshops I run and presentations I give. Some of these are on aspects of reading, writing or crafts; but I also run presentations on life as a disabled person.

Many people want to know more about life with a disability, but don't know how to find out. When giving these presentations, I've encountered newly diagnosed MSers who hope to learn something about what they can expect; there are friends and family of disabled people; disabled people who want to learn how I explain things; medical / service professionals and interested members of the public. I've seen Red Cross volunteers, members of the clergy, people who work in shops, osteopaths and people with specific queries regarding their own disabilities. I don't mind why a person attends, I'm just glad of the chance to demonstrate what being disabled means today.

The talk begins with me making a statement that I have multiple sclerosis, and an explanation that although I speak from my own life, I also draw on the experiences of other disabled people who've confided in me over the years. This allows me to be very honest when answering frank questions, with a lot less embarrassment for all concerned as I don't always specify whether I'm talking about my own experiences or someone else's.

I use a range of props to explain some of the invisible aspects of disability – such as a mains cable with broken insulation to illustrate the damage MS has inflicted on my spinal cord. More interestingly, I have several items that enable some able-bodied attendees to experience the difficulties of being disabled. These include a pair of my old glasses, smeared with petroleum jelly to simulate blurred vision – apparently it's similar to the effect of macular degeneration. I get volunteers to try performing basic tasks whilst using crutches or a wheelchair – such as going through a fire door or filling a bottle with water in the kitchen. I issue several people with surgical-type gloves, to simulate reduced manual sensation and dexterity, then ask them to perform everyday tasks, such as peeling a Satsuma or tying a tie. I confess I get a certain sadistic pleasure from asking ladies from the Women's Institute to knit whilst wearing gloves!

One of my favourite demonstrations is to pick a volunteer who's wearing shoes with noticeable heels. I ask her to remove one shoe and replace it with a swimming flipper. She then has to walk around the room, which isn't too bad – until I ask her a question. This break in concentration is usually enough to make her stumble – which demonstrates beautifully that compensating for as disability may appear easy, but not if you're trying to do something else at the same time! This is an accurate demonstration of a condition called drop foot, which is very common in MS and other neurological illnesses.

These talks have proved quite popular, at least in bookings. Often, a group leader will book me to talk, but a percentage of their membership will happen to have something more important to do that evening. I conclude that the organisers recognise the value of my presentation, but some of their members would prefer not to learn anything about disabilities. This is a real shame, but I suppose it's inevitable. What I'd love to do is present my material to school children, in the hope that they will learn to be more open-minded than some of the older generation.

I usually find there are people who've come along to ask specific questions, perhaps about the correct choice of wheelchair for an aging parent or how to arrange alterations to their home. Other questions that crop up are about the everyday things we take for granted. One lady asked me how I put my socks on – I demonstrated by reaching down for the hem of my jeans and pulling my ankle onto the opposite thigh. (I'm not as flexible as I used to be and have to pull and push my legs into place, but I can still get into lotus position. Just!)

So what do I aim to achieve at a talk? Well, much the same as in this book.

- I try to explain that disabilities aren't always visible, and even when some symptoms can be seen, there may be more that aren't evident.
- I try to demonstrate that it's possible to laugh at aspects of a disability in a shared way, not a cruel one.
- I try to break the taboo that surrounds disability by answering the questions that people have never dared to ask a disabled person before.
- I try to be realistic about the impact of disability on people's lives – neither totally negative nor positive.
- I try to demonstrate the idea that a disability has more implications than are obvious – such as manoeuvring through a fire door in a manual wheelchair.

The vast majority of people who've been to one of these talks respond very positively – often thanking me afterwards for being so open and honest about the problems disabled people face every day. As with any of these talks, the truest test is in the number of repeat bookings I get – and the number of people who couldn't make it the first time finding they're more available!

Much of this may sound trivial and perhaps it is. But as long as I keep getting such positive feedback, I will continue to present these talks.

Let's Shake on That

Let's call him Andy – not his real name.

I knew Andy when I worked in mobile telecommunications. He was based at the opposite end of the country and we'd been communicating by email and phone for years. We'd grown quite friendly – chatting comfortably, flirting a little. You know the sort of thing.

Andy emailed to say he would be coming to our offices for a training course the following week. He suggested meeting up, so we could put a face to each other's names. I agreed readily.

I reached the building where the training course was running just before one o'clock and made my way to the room where they'd have lunch. There were a few people I already knew and I chatted with them for a moment. Then I heard someone say,

"Andy – here's Meg."

I turned to see him and reached out my hand to shake. I saw him reach out automatically, then snatch his hand away with a look of such disgust that I physically recoiled. Everything happened in slow motion; I watched his changing expressions and fought down the nausea in my own stomach. I was new to using a wheelchair at work and couldn't believe how strong a reaction I had provoked. Was I really so disgusting?

Andy muttered a few polite phrases, made his excuses and avoided me for the rest of the visit.

This isn't an isolated example – a significant percentage of people won't shake hands with a person in a wheelchair. Reactions vary from mild discomfort to open disgust, and I have learnt to spot the no-touchers very quickly. I usually take pity and don't even offer my hand – although I have been known to insist on shaking when I want to make a point. I'm most annoyed when it's someone who's being paid to provide me a service and is obviously unwilling to treat me with the same courtesy they would an able-bodied person.

A tutor on a course I attended seemed like the no-touch type, and I tested my perceptions by offering my hand in the course of a conversation. He pointedly didn't shake and I didn't push the point. However, he got caught out later in the week. He proposed an exercise which began with us drawing slips of paper from a hat and someone suggested he use a real hat, since I was wearing one. I agreed readily and my hat was passed along the table towards him. It was clear that he didn't want to touch something I had been wearing – but he couldn't really get out of doing so. He managed to get through the drawing-names-out-of-a-hat part by touching the hat as little as possible – but another person commented to me afterwards that she thought he acted oddly. Nice to know someone else noticed.

There are many people who know me but have never met me – friends as well as people I work with. Many people who know me through the internet don't know I'm disabled (although this book's a bit of a giveaway) and most editors who've published my work don't know. I don't mention my disability unless it's relevant in some way. If I'm writing a report for a disability magazine, it's almost a qualification that I have to state; but if I'm submitting a general-interest item to a mainstream publication, it's not relevant and I don't mention it, any more than my waist-length hair!

Family Gatherings

Funerals are never exactly pleasant occasions. At this particular one I was due to travel in one of the funeral cars, together with my husband and other members of the family. Arriving at the house early, Hubby and I settled on the sofa out of everyone's way. Some relatives arrived unexpectedly and I overheard a snatch of the conversation.

"It's alright – we can make room for you."

I nudged Hubby. "We're about to be pushed out of the car," I whispered.

He didn't have time to answer before another voice cut in.

"Me-eg."

I looked up, knowing what was coming.

"Wouldn't you be better off in your own car? I know you're meant to be in the proper one, but surely it's better to travel in your own."

"No, I'm fine. Funeral cars are designed to be accessible and there'll be plenty of room for my crutches," I replied.

"But you'd be better ...?"

Now what can I say? If I insist on travelling in the funeral car, I'm being awkward on a day when people don't want the hassle. I've already been told not to use my wheelchair "because it'll get in everyone's way" and I don't know how far I'm going to have to struggle on my crutches if I'm not in the official car. I tried to think of a better solution whilst ignoring the repeated assurances that it was best for me. As usual, I chose the easiest solution.

"Okay, we'll take our car."

So, there we were, stuck at the back of the funeral cortège. At the chapel we had to park at the far end of the car park, as the other guests were already inside; and I struggled all the way up their gravelled car park. Likewise at the crematorium and the club where refreshments were provided afterwards. We were stuck at the back and had to walk furthest, a fact which wasn't helped by the number of disabled bays occupied by cars without a badge on display.

So what could I have done? There's no way to insist that I can manage without making a scene nobody wants. I could have decided to use my wheelchair, since I had to walk much further now I'd been pushed to the sidelines, but the chapel and the club weren't properly wheelchair-accessible and there was that gravel car park! I chose to make myself ill by trying to please someone else.

It's possible that people genuinely believe they're doing what's best for me – thinking that they're better able to judge my needs than I am; that I'm just being "noble" by protesting. I try to believe that they mean well, but it's difficult - especially when their idea of helping me happens to coincide with what suits them best. If someone needs to make a sacrifice, it's amazing how often it happens to be the one with the disability.

A conversation on another day. I'd just found out there had been a family party I wasn't invited to.

"We've stopped inviting you because you always make excuses not to go," she said.

"What sort of excuses? Do you mean events I couldn't attend because of the MS?" I asked.

"It's nothing to do with your so-called disability. You just make excuses all the time!"

"So what have I made excuses for that weren't MS-related?" I asked.

"Oh, I can't think of any at the moment. But you do it all the time and you blame your MS when it suits you."

If I try hard enough, I can see how people's perception might lead them to think I use MS as an excuse, but when I think of family events I didn't attend, I have a different view. For example:

The birthday party at a house with a long, gravel path from the nearest parking.

"The toilet's upstairs, but you can manage, can't you?"

The wedding at a venue chosen for its majestic staircase – with no lift up to the function room.

A party on the day after I return home from holiday, exhausted from travelling.

A Civil Partnering at the other end of the country after I've got an unavoidably busy week.

One of the hardest things to explain to people is how these apparently small problems can be enough to leave me ill for a week after everyone else has forgotten I was struggling at all.

On top of the obvious problems with venues, there are lots of minor inconveniences that make any sort of social gathering harder for those of us with mobility problems. Buffets are murder in a wheelchair and even worse on crutches. How do you carry your plate? How do you place anything on it? Is there enough room to get near the table? Then there's the problem of accessible toilets – if there is one, there's a good chance it's on the opposite side of the building from the function rooms. A large number of people getting tipsy and not watching what's behind them is often funny, but downright dangerous if you're in a wheelchair. The list goes on, but I won't!

Some relatives are fine about this. Some people accept me saying "I might attend," understanding that I can't promise anything. Some family members ask what they can do to make it easier for me and genuinely try to help. These people are such a relief after the ones who insist on a firm commitment or tell me they know what I need and then impose their own preferences. Some people who've known me all my life seem determined to insist that they know what's best for me; or they refuse to believe I have a genuine disability.

So, I have a policy of only attending events where I can be reasonably sure it's accessible enough and that I will have the energy to cope with the problems that arise on the day. I've explained this over and over again, but I still get accused of using MS as an excuse. Sometimes I arrange to visit the hosts after an event – at a time when I am able to travel and there aren't as many people around for me to worry about.

Your family are assumed to be the people who stand by you, no matter what life throws at you. The reality is somewhat different. Developing a chronic condition highlights those members of your extended family who truly care about you, whilst some just blame you for being awkward.

I have relatives who've been helpful and understanding in my years of need. On the other hand, some family members highlight the problems caused by my disability in a very negative way. If friends don't respond well to a disability, you move on and make new friends. You don't have that choice with your family.

Returning to Work

Since leaving full-time employment, I sometimes think I might be able to return to the office. It generally happens after a couple of weeks of feeling better than usual. Maybe this is it, maybe I could actually go back to earning a living the way I used to!

I went through a phased return to work several years ago, after major surgery. The idea was that I would start at four hours a day, increasing over the first few weeks until I was back up to a full day. I was also told to phone in and say I was staying at home if I needed to, without taking a day's sick leave. Foolishly, I did not get any of this in writing. From my first day back in the office, I was pressured to work longer hours. The rest of the team were told to take work off me if I was finding it too demanding, which didn't make me popular. I sacrificed things outside of work to keep up with everyone's requirements – I was often too tired to cook a meal; tickets for a show were wasted because I wasn't well enough to go; some days I couldn't even eat a meal when my Hubby got us a take-out. But I did return to work.

For once, I actually learned something from this experience. I decided that if I was going to survive another phased return to work, it would be by my own rules. I would put myself to the test – before I set foot back in the office. I would start by sitting at my PC for two hours every day, starting at nine o'clock prompt. The idea was to simulate something of the working environment and see how I got on. It worked. Not by getting me back to work, but by convincing me that I wasn't able to. It only took three days.

Since then, I have advised other people to try the same. If you're thinking of a return to work after a long-term illness, work out a way to do a trial run.

- Get up at the right time.
- Dress appropriately for your anticipated work.
- Set up a "working environment" – in my case, a desk with a PC on it.
- Decide on a short "working day" – I started with just two hours.
- Start "work" at the same time each day.
- Stick with it for the allocated time, although you're allowed coffee / loo breaks.
- If you smoke, you must go outside to do so – whatever the weather.
- At the end of your time, leave your workstation.
- Remember you still have to do all your other jobs – like childcare, cooking and shopping.
- Do this for a week and see how you feel at the end of it.
- If it's going well, increase your daily hours for the second week.

The advantage of this method is that it allows you to measure your own fitness in the relative comfort and privacy of your own home, instead of going back to work and finding out you aren't well enough. And if you are fit to work, you build up your stamina slowly at the same time as convincing yourself you can do it.

Whether you're returning to work with your previous employer or starting a new job, it's important to be honest with the management. Tell them what you think you can do, discuss a phased start if that's appropriate and make sure everything is put in writing. If it's written down, everyone knows exactly where they stand and what is expected of them. If you're returning to work under a government scheme, this documentation is likely to be written by whoever is helping you return, but it's still a good idea to make sure you've got your own copy, with signatures from all parties.

Retiring on Health Grounds

"Why are you still working, Meg?"

The question came from my manager, just before my annual appraisal. I couldn't answer him then, though I now know why I carried on working as long as I could. It's important for me to feel that I'm doing something worthwhile and that used to mean going into the office, doing my job and knowing my salary hit my bank account every month.

I got my first job at the age of fourteen, serving in a local shop and held a variety of part-time jobs through school and university. I've rarely been out of work and kept myself as busy as I'm able even since "retiring". It's hard to admit you can no longer hold down a "proper" job. This book is evidence that I'm still trying to contribute, even though I'm no longer able to work regular hours. I never made the decision to stop working, my body and my MonSter made it for me.

In the last years of my "normal" working life, my progressive disability interfered more and more with everything I tried to do. I requested adaptations to my working environment and some were implemented. My furniture was adjusted, a printer was located on my desk to save me crossing the office, a bar was fitted to the wall to help me transfer between my wheelchair and desk chair. But other requests were turned down - no funding was available to help buy me a powered wheelchair and the insurance department informed me that they would not allow me to keep one in the office if I paid for it myself. My requests to work from home or reduce my hours were turned down because it wouldn't be fair on everyone else. Under the DDA every employer has a right to refuse any change they feel to be unreasonable, so this is all perfectly legal.

I continued to drag myself into the office. I knew my health was worsening and the management commented on it – but only in terms of my failing to keep it to myself. As long as my work was satisfactory, no-one would consider making significant accommodations for me.

Until the day that I couldn't even get myself out of bed. I phoned in sick. A week later, I saw my GP for the obligatory sick note and was signed off for another couple of weeks. It wasn't until the third sick note that the manager contacted me.

He came to visit. He told me I looked well and asked when I was coming back. I explained that I was still unfit for work and asked again if reduced hours were an option. He said not – if I were allowed to work part-time, other people would insist on it, too. I asked about working from home, but this was refused for the same reason.

The weeks turned into months. I was starting to recover slightly, but still unable to "work" for more than short periods at unpredictable intervals. (I had started to write, in a very limited way.) The manager visited again. This time he suggested I could come back on a part-time basis. He asked if I had broadband available at home, as I might be able to do some of my work from there. He even suggested emailing me some tasks to "see how I got on with it" – while I was still under doctor's orders not to work. I said I would think about all of these points.

I discussed the matter with my GP, who was horrified to hear that I was being pushed into going back to work before she thought I should. She told me to request details of the offered assistance in writing, saying I mustn't even consider restarting work unless I had this written confirmation. I did as she said, but the requested assurances were never provided. Looking back, I think I had a narrow escape. If I'd been foolish enough to go back, the promises could have evaporated as quickly as they were made and the main casualty would have been my health.

Even though I'm not able to work regular hours, there are some jobs that are possible. As well as my writing, I do some mystery shopping, which is an occupation I'd recommend for anyone in my position. It's very flexible and undemanding – but no-one will ever get rich doing it. There are always reputable companies looking to recruit shoppers, both disabled and able-bodied. Like I mentioned at the top of this chapter, it's important to me that I feel I'm doing something worthwhile.

Many of us find it hard to accept that we are no longer fit to work, whether because of reaching retirement age or ill-health. I never really made the decision to retire, and would probably have been healthier if I had stepped down in a more controlled manner. It may have been better for me to have accepted my own limitations, rather than working until I had no choice. But I would probably make the same mistake again.

Being Green

The Green-Eyed Monster

"You're really lucky to be disabled, Meg."

The comment came just like that, without preamble, from another student at the evening classes we were studying. The occasion was an event at a local college; I was in my wheelchair, my husband in close attendance. We were both gobsmacked. We'd struggled to park in the tiny space reserved for blue badge holders and pushed my wheelchair up the ramps to the building. The venue was barely accessible due to ill-placed furniture narrowing doorways and corridors. I couldn't work out what would make someone say such a thing!

"I'm sure you don't mean that," I replied eventually.

"It's so easy for you – you didn't have to walk up that hill from the car park," he replied.

He was entirely serious; believing that the privileges associated with my disability outweighed any minor inconveniences it may cause.

I've heard disability envy expressed in many forms, but none as blunt as that.

He's not alone. I've met many people who are actually jealous of those with disabilities. Somehow they believe that a debilitating condition is a small price to pay for the obvious advantages. I find this incomprehensible. It took me a long time to accept that there are those who think this way, but the conclusion is inescapable.

Disability envy manifests in a variety of ways. Some people believe that being disabled automatically brings me large financial benefits. When I try to explain that this isn't the case, as most benefits are means tested, they can get quite aggressive and often insist that I'm lying as "everybody knows" disabled people get huge amounts of money from the tax payers. I won't debate the politics of the welfare state – but I will say that being disabled does not automatically qualify me for massive payouts. Nor does it make me a sponger, a skiver or a faker.

Then there are the people who see what they think of as preferential treatment for the disabled. Parking bays are a common issue. Contrary to popular thinking, disabled people aren't automatically issued with a blue parking badge; it's only available to those who need it due to severe difficulty in walking, etc. Being able to park close to the entrance of a venue, shop or whatever enables the badge-user to attend an event, go shopping or do anything else a non-disabled person might do. If I always had to park 200 yards away, I wouldn't be able to do *anything*. Believe me, if I had the choice, I would rather park in the main car park and *run*. Disabled parking spaces are often an afterthought and far from being the privilege some people believe, they can be positioned badly without considering the needs of the people who have to use them – quite a few don't have dropped kerbs, for example. Similarly the provision of disabled toilets. They're not some sort of special, luxury bathroom for the privileged few – they're essential for those of us who need extra space, a sink close to hand, etc. and they are often badly maintained. I've ranted elsewhere about able-bodied people who try to justify using disabled facilities, (see Seeing Red). But at least the people who see them as a privilege are jealous of something tangible, however misguided. I've read accounts by disabled sportspeople commenting that some competitors in disabled sports are more able than they claim to be. Once again, these are people who see a real gain to be made from an apparent disability.

The people I find hardest to understand are those who are jealous of the special attention they think disabled people get. I know many people feel sympathy for me because of my disability, but I do *not* take advantage of this and hate to learn that someone actually pities me (shudder!). The few people who've been asked their opinion on some of these chapters are under strict instructions not to see it as a request for sympathy – and to comment only on my writing. I have known people who've pretended to be ill for the sympathy it gets them. There are people who like to be the "needy" one in the group and who see someone with a visible disability as competing for this attention – and resent them for it. I've met individuals who, after recovering from a lengthy illness, claim to be disabled because they've found this can be used to manipulate others to their advantage. I really find this attitude impossible to believe. Sympathy is a fine and very human emotion. I'm as sympathetic as anyone about other people's problems; but telling lies to pressurise people into it? Words fail me.

Disability is something we all have to live with, whether in ourselves or in other people. It's just one facet of our lives and we make our own decisions about how we cope with it. It brings more negatives than positives, both for the disabled person and those around them. It restricts what we can do and often how long we will live. How can anyone be jealous of that?

Disability Etiquette

"I'm selfish, impatient and a little insecure. I make mistakes, I am out of control and at times hard to handle. But if you can't handle me at my worst, then you sure as hell don't deserve me at my best." — Marilyn Monroe

There is a legend about Sir Gawain of Arthur's court going on a quest to find out what it is that all women desire most. He spent a year and a day trying to find the answer – Riches? A strong, handsome husband? Good food and wine? (Author's note: Chocolate?) Fine clothes? To be courted with flowers and jewellery?

A storyteller friend spins this story out for several minutes, but I'll leap to the punch line. A lady wants to make up her own mind. So does a man, for that matter. The same even applies to people with disabilities.

When I present my *Disability Awareness* talk, I'm often asked, "How should I speak to a disabled person?"

There's really only one answer – deal with us as if we're people. Most of us are!

Pardon my sarcasm, but it's true.

If it's any consolation, disabled people can have exactly the same problem. Some of this chapter is about my experiences as a disabled person, as well as ancient history from when I wasn't.

A casting director once told me that she'd just met a young lady who didn't have a right arm and wasn't sure whether to offer a hand to shake. As it happens, I know the person she was talking about and that she'd have accepted the hand by shaking it – with her left hand. If you're uncertain because you've never met someone with that disability before, just remember the other person *does* have experience of meeting able-bodied people!

If someone really isn't able to shake hands, they can decline with a smile, usually appreciating that you've treated them as you would anyone else. I once met a man who couldn't lift either arm to shake, but could bend to kiss my hand. Nice alternative!

The same rule applies to other situations. If I'm talking to a blind person, I still make eye contact. Even if they can't tell, I can! And I treat them exactly as I would a sighted person. If I meet a blind friend in town, I greet him by using his name and mine – "Hi Derek, it's Meg". I don't expect him to recognise my voice and the slightly longer greeting gives him time to work out where I am.

I've learnt that deaf people have different needs for understanding me when I'm speaking to them. I speak a *little* louder if I know someone's hard of hearing, but don't slow down unless I'm asked to. And I'll happily turn my head to give them their preferred angle for lip-reading if prompted. I know enough BSL (the alphabet and some useful words) to spell out anything I'm not saying clearly enough.

People with mental health problems– and some without - often don't like to be touched and prefer not to shake hands. I still offer, but watch for signs that they'd rather not. This ain't rocket surgery (to use my favourite mixed metaphor).

Back in the days before I needed walking aids myself, I would make eye contact with anyone who looked as if they may need assistance – such as a wheelchair user in a supermarket. It only takes a little smile to tell them you're happy to help if they need it. I still do the eye contact thing, although I'm not very good at reaching things from high shelves any more.

Okay, it doesn't always work. There have been times when someone mistakes my friendly smile as an invitation to tell me all their woes. In great detail. And I've had "What are you staring at?" thrown at me. But it doesn't put me off. Surprising though it may sound, people with disabilities are not all the same and some of us can be selfish, grumpy or easily offended. Funny that – you'd think we were almost human!

The astute reader will have noticed that I keep using the word *offer*. In my experience, most people prefer help to be offered rather than assumed. Just as some women are offended by a man holding a door open for them, some disabled people (myself included) may not be grateful if you assume you know what we want and do it without asking. This isn't about being brave or independent – sometimes you can make things harder by insisting that you help.

There are common misconceptions about "political correctness": that it is always a bad thing and that it's simply a case of not using certain words. I think it's simply common courtesy and more to do with intentions than specific terminology. Some disabled people dislike the word *handicapped*, as it's derived from the term *cap-in-hand* and implies that disabled people are beggars. But if people don't know the history of the word, is it fair to object to them using it? I pay more attention to how someone speaks to me than the words they use. I will correct people if their use of medical terminology could cause problems, such as describing me as *wheelchair bound* when they mean *wheelchair user*, or *she's in a wheelchair*. I can stand up, and even manage a few steps with assistance, so I'm not bound to my wheelchair. Political correctness does cause problems if people are too scared to use an honest word or phrase – but common courtesy is unlikely to offend.

When asked, "How should I describe you?" I invariably answer, "My name is Meg, my hair is waist-length and my eyes are green." I know that's not what they mean, but I don't think my disability is the only thing needed to describe me. Some disabled people describe themselves in the harshest of terms, encouraging others to do the same. I'm not sure the term *spastic* can ever be used affectionately, whether the person has cerebral palsy or not. But I will fight for anyone's right to choose what they call themselves!

I've also heard people stumble when they've said something that they think might be offensive. I don't think many wheelchair users will object to someone saying, "Let's walk over there." I've never heard a blind person complain when someone says, "See you tomorrow." Worrying about such comments really is taking political correctness too far!

If you're trying to see a situation from a disabled person's view, it's easy to think you understand more than you do. In conversation with a friend, I said,

"Have you ever been on a train in a wheelchair?"

"No, but I've taken my Mother-in-Law by train," he replied. "You get treated like royalty, with people waiting to help you off and everything."

Well, usually true. But in that situation, the person in the wheelchair obviously had an able-bodied helper with her, which makes a huge difference. Those same people once helped me onto my connecting train and left me there for forty minutes until it pulled out. I couldn't leave as they'd taken the ramp, there wasn't an accessible loo and I didn't know what was going on. That's the difference between helping someone and living through something yourself. Similarly, taking a child somewhere in a pushchair is not the same as being in a wheelchair. You can lift the child up a 5" kerb – I can't lift my wheelchair up the same height. I'm not criticising – but there's a huge gap between observing and experiencing. Yes, you can get some small idea of a disability at one remove, just as my own extreme short-sightedness gives me the tiniest taste of the effect blindness has on a person – but it's important to realise how far your own experiences fall short of actual disability.

I heard a news report on radio recently, where a woman with early-onset Parkinson's disease commented that she finds it very difficult to walk, but can run far more comfortably. I was impressed with her candour and have a lovely mental image of people watching her struggle to walk and their amazement when she breaks into a trot. I wish I was as able to shock people who make similar assumptions about my disability!

When we meet someone, we're likely to focus on their differences, on what makes them unlike us. This isn't necessarily all "bad" if it means we're more likely to offer help. But it's better to focus on our similarities. I appreciate this can be difficult, but I can assure you we're all human inside. Personally, I prefer people to see what I can do, rather than what I can't. But the important thing is to give a disabled person the chance to accept or decline help, as they prefer – just as you would yourself.

Last year, I'd been upset by someone who'd been lecturing me on how difficult my presence was making things for other people. Someone else, Colin, noticed my tears and crouched next to my chair to ask what was wrong. I just told him it was because of some unkind remarks and didn't elaborate. But I appreciated his empathy – and the hug.

When I next saw Colin, he seemed a little uncomfortable.

"I'm sorry to ask, but did you mind me coming down to speak to you?" he asked.

"Erm, no," I answered.

"Only I was afraid it looked a bit, well, patronising."

I couldn't help but smile. "Not at all. It's lovely when people make the effort like that."

It's a shame that I mention this event as being unusual. Some people try to be helpful, but it's rare anyone actually asks if they're doing the right thing.

And I'm a woman who appreciates being asked.

Vegboxes and Delivery Men

Shopping is a pleasure that becomes a chore when you don't drive, can't carry much, don't fit into changing rooms and tire easily. Days of tramping around a shopping centre with a growing collection of carrier bags are suddenly difficult to the point of impossibility. Much of my shopping is now done by post, phone or over the internet, leaving me with the energy to do the fun bits in person.

Supermarket shopping on the internet has become easy, efficient and cheap. True, there are some things you'd rather select in person, but online shopping is a good way to buy all the heavy, bulky items. Even the supermarkets that don't offer a full web-shopping option will sometimes deliver – our local one allows customers to shop in person and leave their shopping at the store for delivery the same day, including chilled and frozen items.

I get a vegbox delivered to my doorstep once a week. This service has matured well from its early beginnings; customers now have good control over the items they receive. I use one that offers a selection of boxes, with their contents listed on the website each week; so I can choose the most appropriate one. Got visitors coming to stay? Order a larger box. Don't want potatoes? Choose a spud-free box. Want a specific item? Order it as an extra. This particular company also offers meat, dairy products and store cupboard essentials, so it's a really useful service. The fruit and veg are significantly cheaper than the supermarkets and sourced as locally as possible, cutting back on food miles for those who care about the environment.

It's often said that mail-order companies are killing the High Street. This may be true, but it's difficult to browse a small bookstore from a wheelchair and most clothing stores have miniscule changing rooms, so it can be easier to buy books online and order clothes from a company that offers free delivery and returns. I still shop at local shops when I can, but I have to be practical about my limitations.

There are some excellent online deals for larger purchases, too. I'm more likely to buy electrical goods over the internet than in a shop, though I like to actually try furniture before purchase.

I use a cashback service for much of my web shopping. These are great. For the uninitiated, if you click on an advert for a website, the advertiser receives a kickback from the company you then buy from. Cashback sites collect the same kickback, but pass it back to the purchaser. On occasions, I've received more than 10% of the purchase price in this way, on top of other discounts. Useful for large purchases such as a new washing machine, holidays, pressies and lots of other things.

My favourite way to enjoy an occasional day's shopping from a wheelchair is to get my husband to drop me at our local indoor shopping centre. I can easily get round as the floors are level, tiled and well-served by lifts. I don't have to carry much, as I've already ordered most things for home delivery. There's a nice big bookshop with helpful staff who are never too busy to pass me a book from the top shelf. Numerous cafes and food outlets offer opportunities for a leisurely bite or a coffee whilst watching the world go by. I have a large bag that fits on the back of my chair, allowing me to carry a lot before I start slinging bags over the handles and on my lap. I even know which clothes shops have large enough changing rooms for me to use. By the time Hubby comes back, he collects a tired, burdened and impoverished shopper with a big smile on her face.

Mail order shopping can be much easier and cheaper than a trip to the shops, but it will never completely replace the browsing experience.

The down side of mail order is usually at the delivery end. To me, an item is delivered when it's handed to the purchaser. To certain delivery companies; it's delivered when they dump it in your garden. This has happened too many times to count and I have complained on many occasions. If I've ordered boxes of wine and they've been left in the back garden, I may have to get a neighbour to carry them in for me. Which costs me a bottle of wine (to thank him) when I've supposedly already paid for delivery. I've had food deliveries left in the dustbin and one delivery company even thought it was appropriate to force the garage door open to leave a parcel inside. All of these things can happen to any shopper, but it's doubly difficult for the disabled person to manage. The most worrying trend I've noticed is in preconceptions about disabled people among certain delivery drivers. One driver in particular always spoke very slowly to me, as if I were either deaf or stupid. When he delivered a box that had clearly been opened and some of the contents removed, I phoned the depot to complain. The lady who spoke to me suggested that I might be "confused" over the number of items I'd ordered and refused to look for them at the depot. I suspect that other disabled or elderly people get bullied by this kind of service and even come to accept the losses it causes. It's a sorry world where vulnerable people are seen as easy victims for thieves working in the service industry, but it obviously happens.

Public Transport

It's rare to find users of the UK public transport system who have a good word to say about it. Unreliability, delays, poor co-ordination of services, the wrong sort of leaves on the line – the list is endless. It's unlikely these obvious problems will be resolved in the immediate future, which might explain why making the service accessible for the disabled is not a priority.

Some years ago, the major bus company that serves the city I lived in proudly announced that a quarter of their buses were now wheelchair accessible. Just think about that for a moment – it means that three-quarters were not wheelchair-friendly. So, a wheelchair user could expect to watch three buses go past before one arrived that they could use. And this was something to boast about! Many railway stations are not accessible – I can only reach one platform at my local station, as the other one is only accessible via a footbridge. So I can get on a train going east, but going west means a detour. (I get on an east-bound train, get off at the next station, wheel myself out of the station and across the road to the other platform.) Strangely, this is exacerbated by increased safety regulations. Staff used to be allowed to take a wheelchair across the line by means of a "barrow crossing" between the rails, but this isn't permitted now - it's considered too dangerous. And me wheeling over a level crossing is *safe?*

Despite this, travelling by train is the best way for someone in a wheelchair. People who need assistance can book it in advance, (get the phone number for your Rail Operator's *assistance service* from National Rail Enquiries). Staff at stations and on the trains are almost always helpful and there's generally someone waiting with a ramp to assist me on and off the train. Intercity trains usually have accessible toilets close to designated wheelchair spaces. In other words, it should be a delight. Unfortunately, a percentage of passengers resent disabled people getting "special" treatment. The space designated for wheelchairs is often full of pushchairs, large cases, cycles and whatever. Staff will sometimes remove these items to make room for me to park, but their owners may complain – to me, after the guard's moved on. People travelling with young children have insisted they have "a right" to use wheelchair-designated spaces and it's me who should go somewhere else. My only defence is to point out I *can't* go anywhere else, whilst they have the choice.

My preferred method is to park my wheelchair in the reserved space and transfer onto a normal seat. A wheelchair isn't designed to give good support on a moving vehicle and the brakes certainly aren't designed to cope with the acceleration and braking. But leaving my wheelchair unoccupied carries other risks.

I've seen muddy cycles placed deliberately on my wheelchair, as if it's a convenient bike-park. One man dropped his large, heavy suitcase onto the footplate, lifting the rear wheel off the floor (which means the brakes are unconnected). I've even seen someone remove my bag and sit in the wheelchair themselves – when there were plenty of other seats available.

The assistance provided by rail staff is usually very good, although you sometimes need to shout loudly to make sure someone comes to help. I've had a few near-misses, but thankfully no repeats of my worst-ever trip.

I was travelling from Chepstow in South Wales to a station on the North Wales coast, a journey which is complicated as there is no direct line. I had to catch a train from Chepstow to Newport (travelling West); from there to Gloucester (going North-East), then one to Machynlleth

(North-West) and finally a slower train that follows the scenic coastal route.

The problem came at Gloucester.

I had made myself known to the Train Manager, who'd double-checked that I was getting off at Gloucester and said she'd phone ahead to make sure they were ready for me. The train pulled into Gloucester station and I positioned myself near the exit, baggage loaded onto the back of my wheelchair. The other passengers got off, new ones came on and I was still sitting in the open doorway. I had seen a man wandering around with the ramp but had failed to attract his attention.

Then the door closed in front of me.

I wasn't sure what to do. I thought about pulling the emergency cord, but it was out of reach and while I was thinking the train began to move. With me still aboard.

Now, even on accessible trains, there isn't room for a wheelchair to pass along the aisle, so I couldn't go anywhere in search of assistance. I returned to the wheelchair space and persuaded another passenger to go in search of the train manager. He came back in three minutes, saying he'd found her and she'd promised to come straight down. Actually, it was almost fifteen minutes later.

"Mrs Kingston, isn't it?" she asked.

"Yes, hello. What's happening?" I replied.

"You didn't get off the train."

"Well, er, no. The ramp wasn't brought," I explained.

"Are you sure?" she asked.

That struck me as an odd question. "Quite sure. I saw someone with a ramp, but he didn't come near the door I was waiting at."

"Did you try to get his attention?"

"Well, yes. But there's not much I can do from inside the train." Believe me, Reader, there isn't.

"Hm, so you didn't do anything. It's their responsibility to get you off," she carefully wasn't meeting my eye.

"I don't actually care whose responsibility it is. What do I do now?"

"You'll have to get off at the next station," she said.

"And that is...?"

"Crewe. We can't stop any earlier and let you off."

And she walked away before I could say any more.

We didn't see a member of train staff for the rest of our journey to Crewe. The passengers who'd got on at Gloucester didn't have their tickets checked so it's possible a few had a free ride. I don't know!

At Crewe, there were two members of staff waiting, with ramp, at the point where I would get off. They put the ramp in place and waited while I rolled down it.

"Hello. Can you tell me what I need to do next?" I asked.

"Come with us," replied one of the men.

They walked away and left me to follow them across the station to the customer services. One of them disappeared as we arrived, the other went through a door labelled, "Staff Only" and shut it behind him. After several minutes, I joined the queue for service, as he didn't seem to be coming back. It took another few minutes before the same man appeared. He handed me a sheet of paper, saying,

"Here's your new times."

"Hang on," I replied. This time I was ready for him and grabbed his arm as he turned away.

"This will get me there two hours late."

"That's the next train," he said.

I looked at the itinerary printed on the paper. It listed a train back from Crewe to Gloucester and the remainder of my journey as booked, two hours later.

"I'm sorry, but that's not good enough," I told him.

There followed a farce with me insisting that I wasn't prepared to arrive two hours late, as I'd booked the proper assistance and it was their mistake that had caused the problem. I refused to be intimidated by the increasing number of staff insisting that I had no choice and continued to throw my toys (and anything else I could reach) out of the metaphorical pram. I stuck to the "rules" of good complaining (see page 257) and, eventually, they acquiesced.

Two members of staff escorted me to the taxi rank. They conferred with a driver and left me to be loaded aboard and driven to my destination station. I asked the driver if he could drop me at the conference centre, but he insisted he had to take me to the station stated on my rail ticket – even though he drove past the conference centre to get there. The taxi's meter was running for the whole journey, clocking up just over £175.

At the station, he unloaded my wheelchair from the boot, putting my luggage back on the handles before pushing the chair into position for me to scramble in. It wasn't until after he had driven away that I took the bag off to get my book out and saw the damage. I'm not sure how, but the bag's seam had been ripped open for about 6".

When I got home (via an uneventful train journey!), I phone the Rail Enquiries line to ask how to claim for the damaged bag. The lady I spoke to listened to a few details, interrupting several times and eventually said,

"You can't claim from us."

"Sorry? Why not?"

"You'll have to take it up with the taxi firm. It was obviously him who broke your bag."

"But I don't even have his contact details. It was the rail staff who arranged it..."

"Don't you think you've had enough from us already?"

She hung up.

In the two years since that journey, I've travelled by rail on many occasions, usually on my own. On the vast majority of occasions, the assistance I requested has been provided cheerfully and without problem. There have been difficulties and other passengers have even stood in doorways to prevent the doors closing when staff failed to get me off a train, but I haven't had a repeat journey to Crewe!

There has been another occasion when I contacted a rail company to ask about claiming for damages, though. This time it was a cardigan I'd ruined when I had to push myself up and down steep, cobbled paths to get to the appropriate platform when I hadn't been advised I needed to arrive at a different one. The member of staff who worked at the station refused to help me, walking in front of me along the path and leaving me to struggle. When I phoned to ask how to claim for the damage, I was told that I could not claim as I'd torn the cardigan myself. Whereas the damage would not have happened if I'd been helped along the path by the station staff.

On average, I'd say that train assistance works about 80% of the time.

Being recompensed for damage caused by the actions or inactions of rail staff and their sub-contracted taxi drivers *fails* 100% of the time. In my experience to date.

The Power of Thought

In a world where medical treatment is dominated by drugs and surgery, it's unfashionable to talk about the power of the mind in medicine. Anyone who admits to using relaxation techniques to cope with pain or will-power to fight fatigue is more likely to be called a hippy than respected for managing their symptoms without medical intervention.

Conspiracy theorists complain that drug companies and doctors deliberately promote a negative view of cost-free treatments. I don't believe this– I think they're simply so focussed on what they can prescribe that they don't stop to consider the simpler alternatives.

The press love to report situations where people shut out pain or achieve something they wouldn't have thought possible. You don't have to look as far as a woman miraculously lifting a car off her toddler - you've done it yourself. Think not? How about *Waiting Room Syndrome?* Ever arrived at the dentist's surgery because of toothache, only to have the pain vanish as you walk in the door? You haven't taken any more painkillers, you haven't had any treatment yet – the only thing that could have mustered your body's resources in this way is your own mind.

A young man I used to work with broke his fibula in a paragliding accident. That's the outer bone in your lower leg. He limped down the hill, drove home and carried on as if nothing had happened. It was a few days before he went for an x-ray and learned of the damage. As soon as he knew, he was in far more pain and could hardly walk on it. So why hadn't it been hurting so much beforehand?

After a drugs trial I was involved in, one patient was horrified to learn that he'd been on the placebo and the improvements in his condition were not due to the drug being trialled. He insisted they must be wrong – that he'd been given the proper drug by mistake and wanted to keep receiving it.

The only medical term for the power of the mind to control symptoms is the *placebo effect*. But this sounds really negative, as if we're being fooled into thinking a sugar pill will work. But look at it the other way round. If you can reduce your symptoms by simply thinking you can, why aren't you doing it all the time?

Tests show that branded tablets are more effective than unbranded or shop's own-label ones. This doesn't make sense, as it's exactly the same drug; but somehow we trick our symptoms into responding differently. There have even been a few studies into the effects of different placebos. These have proved that two small tablets are more effective than one large one – but a very small one is better still. In Australia, a drug called Obecalp is sold. It's just a sugar pill and you'll notice it's the word *placebo* spelt backwards. But it can be very effective if the patient believes it will be.

So, I repeat: if our minds are this good at reducing our symptoms without any help, why aren't we doing it all the time?

Perhaps a better term to use is the *power of positive thinking*. That sounds less like snake oil from a quack doctor, but it still has those flower-power connotations. I think of it as a pushing away – instead of focussing on pain, I shove it to one side and think about something else. It does work, however strange it sounds.

On a larger scale, I believe that my refusal to give in to MS helps a lot with my ability to live with it. Whenever a medical professional tells me I should take things easy or stop doing something that's getting difficult for me, my backbone stiffens and I try even harder to do it. It's my Welsh blood – we're a notoriously stubborn race! The trick is to balance this determination against the realities of my condition; to do as much as I can without making my symptoms worse. Of course, I sometimes get it wrong, and pay the price of overdoing things. But that's part of being alive.

It's not just pain, either. Relaxation techniques are reported to help lower blood pressure and reduce symptoms of many long-term conditions. I don't know of any proper studies that have been conducted into these, but I do believe that the effects are real. (Proper medical studies cost a lot of money to run and no-one is going to invest in researching a treatment they can't make a profit from. This is where conspiracy theories begin!) As for stress-related illnesses - there's little doubt that learning to relax properly can help.

There is even evidence that our thoughts influence the way we age. People who have more control over their environment, more independence and better motivation live longer, happier lives than those who don't have those things. Even the smallest detail can help – like being allowed to choose the new wallpaper or having access to a kitchen to make a cuppa, rather than one being provided. Taking the easy option may not be the best way to go!

So how can you use these techniques?

Relaxation. A simple technique that can be meditation, prayer or simply "emptying your mind". Whether you regard it as a religious discipline or not, there is plenty of evidence to support this approach for coping with all kind of problems, from severe pain to mental health issues. Want to try it? Set aside ten minutes a day, perhaps when you get home from work or before you make dinner. Sit comfortably in a room where you won't be disturbed. If you're not of a religious nature, focus on a simple image like a quiet pool of water; don't force it, but let it expand to fill your mind's eye. Sit still for a few minutes. Once you find yourself getting restless, open your eyes, have a good stretch and get on with your day. Do it daily for a couple of weeks and you'll relax for longer each time until you find your own natural rhythm. If you feel better, keep doing it!

Pain Control. To put it simply, don't think about the fact you're in pain. That's about as helpful as telling someone not to think about elephants – because they immediately have a whole herd parading across their mind. So think about something else. With pain, I visualise it as something solid, something real – which I then push into a corner where I don't have to look at it. Once it's a bit further away, I focus on something else and find it's much easier to ignore the beast. Cheaper than painkillers!

If you read this and say, "She doesn't know what she's talking about. She wouldn't be so dismissive if she had my pain", then I agree. *In part.* I don't have your pain, no more than you have mine. Trigeminal neuralgia is meant to be the worst pain a human body can suffer and it's certainly worse than anything else I've known. I can't dismiss it using these techniques, but they *help* and that's what matters.

Okay, I've spent a whole chapter promoting the use of mind over matter and suggesting it *can be* a better solution than drugs. I'm not suggesting we can burn our prescriptions and manage without any formal treatment from the doctor. But maybe we can use less. Certain techniques can be used by anyone, regardless of their medical condition. Pain tolerance can be as effective against a headache as trigeminal neuralgia. And I don't care if you call me a hippy!

Things I Wish Someone Had Told Me
Warning: Slightly icky details.

There are a number of secondary problems arising from my disability that no-one warned me about, until I mentioned that I suffered with them.

I suspect this happens a lot. Those who know about inevitable side effects of a chronic illness don't bother to tell those of us who don't know. Or maybe they expect someone else to tell us. So here are a few pointers that might be useful to others. Some only apply to MSers, but a few are relevant to anyone with a disability.

Foot problems. Human feet have evolved over many years into effective walking platforms, but they are prone to all sorts of problems if they're not looked after properly. Unfortunately for people with neurological problems, it's very difficult to look after something that you can't feel properly and don't use very much. If I'd thought about it, I might have realised I was likely to not notice athlete's foot, a viral wart or an ingrowing toenail. I've now got into the habit of checking my feet regularly - I'll need to get someone else to do it as I get less flexible. I believe it's usual for diabetics to have their feet checked regularly, but not everyone whose far appendages are in danger from their condition.

Constipation. I did warn you about icky details! It's very simple: if you spend all day sitting or lying down, you will get constipated. Doctors tend to prescribe various treatments that can reduce the impact or unblock the system when necessary, but it's best to manage it with diet as far as possible. I recommend lots of water, fresh fruit and veg and a few spoons of hemp seeds every day. Prevention is far better than cure!

Pernicious anaemia. One for the MSers. MS stops the body from digesting vitamin B12 from food. Without B12, your blood cannot make use of the iron you've eaten. Therefore, MSers are likely to suffer from anaemia that doesn't get any better, even if you take iron tablets. So if you're feeling tired (like the MS fatigue wasn't bad enough), ask for a quick blood test. Easily diagnosed, easily treated.

Infections. As well as the odd ways in which illnesses and the immune system interact, there is a problem for anyone who doesn't get out much. If you don't get exposed to other people's bugs, your immune system will get lazy. When I was still working in the office, I was usually the last one to go down with a cold – or didn't catch it at all. Nowadays, I catch anything my Hubby brings home far too easily. And anything viral will result in my MonSter playing up for a week or so once I've fought the bugs off. The medical profession seem to think anyone with a disability is immune-compromised (which we may be) and they tend to pounce on me with vaccinations for this year's flu or anything else that might help. Sometimes I let them. Sometimes I've had enough of feeling like a pin cushion.

Contact lenses. This is an odd one. I've got really poor eyesight and have needed glasses all of my life, although I didn't get them until I was 10. I first bought contact lenses when I was 18 – hard ones in those days, gas permeables in more recent years. From the start I found them easy to wear for as much as 20 hours at a stretch. And then, suddenly, my MonSter decided I couldn't wear them any more. Not even the soft ones. I'm back to glasses again, although I do try putting my contact lenses in every now and again. Just in case the MonSter's relented. I've asked several medical people about this. They all said it's not a recognised problem with MS – but that other MSers have said the same.

Allergies. Another one that doesn't seem to be officially classed as a symptom of MS, but I notice my food allergies have got worse since my MonSter moved in. Hay fever, too. I don't know why, but I know other people have the same problem.

Healing. Cuts and other injuries take longer to heal if you're not active. A bruise is, essentially, a pool of used blood lying under the skin, which heals gradually (and colourfully) over a few days. Most people are aware that bruises take longer to heal as we get older. But for someone with a disability, different parts of their body heal at different rates – almost as if some parts are older than others. In my own case, my hands and arms heal much faster than my legs and feet. For example, if I've fallen in a way that causes bruises on both arms and legs (usually on the stairs), then the bruises on my arms will disappear in about half the time it takes for the ones on my legs to vanish. An odd situation, but not dangerous in any way.

Relearning Skills

In common with many other disabilities, MS often affects a person's dexterity. From the earliest days of my MS symptoms, I have reduced feeling and control of left hand; later the same problem affected my right. As with all of my symptoms, it's never entirely vanished – but I've managed to retain limited use of my hands. So far.

As many readers won't have experienced the effect MS has on sensation, I'll try to explain. The usual description is to say that it's a bit like pins and needles – which is true, but a long way short of the reality. My hands aren't numb, but my sense of touch is altered. If I touch something hot enough to burn, it takes longer for the message to travel along the nerves to my brain than it would in a person with normal neurological function. In other words, I burn myself on the oven door more often than I used to. I can barely feel the wool wrapped around my fingers for knitting and it's hard for me to judge how hard I'm gripping something. As for dexterity, my fingers sort of do what I've told them to, but there's an unpredictable delay between sending the order and it being received, as it were. This is most noticeable when I'm doing something that involves both hands, as one will respond faster than the other. So I try to type the word "welcome" and it comes out as "wleocme". You'll note that I usually correct these typos – through a well-trained spellchecker and careful editing. If any have still slipped through, please accept my apologies.

It's easy to see how these hand problems affect craft activities. When the MonSter first affected my right hand, I gave up on everything crafty, assuming I wouldn't be able to do it. But I started getting bored! My Nana taught me to knit when I was only four and it's a difficult habit to break after all those years. I started again, using thick wool and chunky needles to get around my dexterity problems. I found my index finger wouldn't wrap the wool round the needle properly (apologies to any non-knitters who don't know the jargon) so I experimented with using my middle finger instead. This worked much better and I'm now knitting almost as fast as I used to. Having cracked the problem, I've kept knitting and believe that it helps to keep my hands nimble. There are times when I have real trouble keeping my tension even, so I go back to chunky knitting; but when my hands behave, I can manage shaped socks in 4-ply wool.

There are compromises to be made in the kitchen, too. I take longer to chop an onion than I used to, and it's not as even as it used to be, but does that really matter? My bread rolls are likely to be different sizes and somewhat irregular in shape – but that just means a guest can pick a larger one if they like my home-made bread, and I'll have a smaller one to keep the balance. Neatness is over-rated!

Of course, it's also more dangerous for me to use sharp objects, as my hands are more likely to slip and I can't feel when I cut myself. So I just take a little more care and buy sharp knives with chunkier handles, to reduce the chances of slippage. I'm also more inclined to have gadgets that do some of the cutting for me.

Similarly with other crafts. I'm never going to be able to work really fine embroidery, but I can manage tapestry and cross-stitch passably well. Though I never used to need a needle-threader. With a little ingenuity and compromise between me and my MonSter, I've found I can still do most of the creative things I used to do. If it takes a little longer and it's not as neat as it used to be – I just don't worry about it.

I don't think I'll ever be able to play a musical instrument again – the co-ordination necessary between fingers, lips and lungs is more than I can manage. I can't even beat a regular rhythm on a drum any more. And don't ask about my singing voice!

So some skills I have managed to relearn. I can type and knit, albeit slower than I used to. I can cook, but I can't do things as neatly as I used to. I think making music is beyond me now – but it could be a lot worse. I'm sure my guests appreciate my onion soup, however uneven the slicing, and the bread rolls taste as good as ever.

Call Me Oracle

"What have you done?" I asked, surprised to see a colleague on crutches, his lower leg hidden by a plaster cast.

"A little accident go-karting," he admitted.

"Ouch! Is it broken?"

He nodded, "Badly. I'm gonna be in this cast for months."

We chatted for a while, then I said,

"If you need advice on how to do anything on crutches, just ask."

He thought for a moment, suddenly went bright red and looked away. It took me a moment to work out what was wrong. A man on crutches has certain difficulties that we women don't have to deal with!

After many years of decreasing physical abilities, I have become something of an expert of how to manage everyday tasks when my hands are on crutches or pushing myself in a wheelchair. Many little things that aren't obvious to someone who hasn't been in that situation. For example, it's not easy to lean on crutches, pull a door towards you and walk through without stumbling. Trust me – I've made a spectacle of myself more than once! Add in the need to swipe a security card before pulling the door and it starts to feel as if you need to be an octopus.

Rather than trying to explain the various little tricks I use, I recommend that anyone who finds themselves in a similar position should take a little time to think it through. There may be a way to do things if you stop and look at the situation. Ask a friend to help you work it out, but choose carefully - it needs to be someone who accepts your abilities as well as your disability.

A few useful tips for the mobility impaired:

- If you're pulling a door towards you when in a wheelchair, you could also be pulling yourself through the door.
- Be prepared to make more trips, carrying less each time.
- If you can't carry it, can you put it on something wheeled and push it? Office chairs are great for shifting PCs around.
- Elbow crutches will stay where they are if you lean your forearm on them, freeing your hand until you need to take a step.
- Like a horse, I have different "gaits" when using crutches. The order in which I move my "four legs" depends on how tired I am, how quickly I want to move and how safe the floor is!
- Lots of tasks can be done sitting down, freeing your hands from the crutches.
- Think about carrying a shoulder bag. The simplest way to free your hands for walking.
- Be prepared to accept help if it's offered. Pride be damned!

With a little thought and practice, many tasks are possible for the person on crutches / in a wheelchair / whatever. Similarly, solutions can be found for problems caused by other disabilities that I don't know.

Because of the gradual way my mobility was worsened, there was never a point when someone suggested I see a physiotherapist for coaching. I keep thinking I should ask for a referral now – but I suspect I know more than they would.

I'm often approached by people asking me how I do something, where I bought a particular aid or if I've come across a particular difficulty. I'm happy to help (unless I'm in a real hurry) and like to think I've made tiny improvements to a lot of lives. Likewise, I sometimes see someone else with a particular way of doing something that I adopt myself. The more we can help each other, the better. After all, who knows better than the person who copes with a disability all the time?

Disability v Disability

We all compare ourselves to others. Whether we feel positive about ourselves – *I'm the brightest in the class; I'm a better runner than him;* or negatively – *I wish I had her figure; I'm always last!* People with long-term conditions are no different and some of us compete over disability itself.

Now, I'd better be honest about this from the start. I try not to compare any disability to another – mine included. Frankly, I don't see what good it does and I'd rather spend my energy fighting my MonSter than measuring it. First of all, it isn't possible to judge a disability – you **can't** know how badly someone else is affected. And how do you judge anyway? My refusal to argue is often seen as an admission that my own disability isn't very serious and I won't defend myself because I know I'd "lose". Ho-hum!

There are some very obvious lines that can be used to divide the disabled community. One is the physical / mental disability split. I've been told, "Physical disability is easier than mental – all you have to do is take more painkillers." I've also heard, "All you have to do with mental problems is to take more anti-depressants." Neither of these is true and, in my view, the comparison doesn't make sense.

One separation that isn't so obvious is between, "Those who are born disabled, those who earn disability and those who have disability thrust upon them." Sorry, Shakespeare. There are some who believe that their disability is worse because they have always had it, whereas those who've become disabled may think their situation is harder because they know what it's like to be able-bodied. This particular debate is further complicated when there's a suggestion that someone caused their own disability –in an accident when they were driving, for example. Once again, I ask - what is the point to this argument? The disabled community suffers enough discrimination from non-disabled people, why do we discriminate amongst ourselves, too?

Even within illnesses, the degree of disability varies tremendously. Take MS as an example. On the one hand, you have the author Michael Crichton, who was diagnosed with MS after a single attack when he was a medical student – and had no further symptoms for the rest of his life. Compare with Jacqueline du Pre, the internationally-renowned cellist, whose MS progressed rapidly and fatally within a few years. Most of us MSers sit somewhere on that spectrum – from those who may have been given a false diagnosis to those whose MonSter attacks quickly and without remission. There are equally large variations in conditions where the diagnosis cannot be disputed, such as people whose prenatal development was impaired by Thalidomide. That drug caused some babies to be born with terrible deformities, without a hope of ever walking or being able to look after themselves; whereas other, more fortunate, victims are able to lead an almost-normal life.

The impact of a disability goes far beyond the immediate effect on the individual who has it. One of the worst aspects is the possibility of children inheriting a condition - a major worry for many disabled people. Whether their condition affected them from birth or developed later, it's something that needs to be taken into account by would-be parents whose disability can be inherited. Sometimes a disability doesn't appear until after they're already a parent and they have to face the fact that it may have been passed on to the next generation without anyone knowing.

Being human, we all respond differently to these challenges. I've known people who cope with the most appalling disabilities, getting on with their life as best they can – often with a shrug and a smile. I've also met people who respond to their diagnosis by labelling themselves as Disabled-with-a-capital-D and almost giving up completely. Not to mention the ones who look for someone to sue and claim every benefit they ever hear of – whether they're entitled to it or not. Okay, my own bias is showing here!

The UK government are now assessing benefit claimants' *abilities*, rather than their disabilities. The idea is to establish what someone is *able* to do, instead of writing them off because of a long-term health condition. Of course, there have been problems with this, as with any system, but the principle is close to my own philosophy – I worked for many years with worsening symptoms and continue to do what I can as a writer and other roles, even though I'm no longer able to work regular hours. I prefer to focus on what I can do, rather than mourn the things I can't.

There are occasions when there is a genuine need to measure someone's disability. This may be an official scale to determine entitlement to benefits or compensation, or the Paralympics Committee drawing up categories to level the playing field for each competitor. In these cases, we can only hope the comparisons are made fairly, without deception or bias on either side.

I'm not in any way disparaging anyone's disability or suffering – merely trying to document the variations that exist under the umbrella term, "disability". From the outside, all disabled people may look alike, but there are as many shades of disability as anything else. None of us can truly measure another's difficulties, only try to empathise.

Doctors – The Manual

Doctors are an essential part of medical care, but how many of us really get the best we can from these useful professionals? This chapter contains many of the tips I've learned over the years.

Note: Throughout, I use the term "doctor" – which could mean your GP, hospital specialist, nurse, osteopath or any other medical practitioner.

Get to Know Your Doctor

No, I'm not suggesting you take him out for a pint, but it's worth paying attention to him as a human being and finding things you have in common. One of "my" doctors used to play rugby – so a rugby analogy will always strike a chord. Not to mention references to drinking and misspent youth. Whatever you find, remember your doctor is a human being, not just a robot that writes prescriptions.

Take a List

Ever walked out of the consulting room to think, "I forgot to ask..."? No? Then you're better organised than I used to be!

If you want to be sure you mention everything, write it down beforehand. I'm **not** suggesting your doctor should help with several ailments each visit – an appointment is for one problem only. But make sure you mention all your relevant symptoms. If you want to give him a lot of information, it's a good idea to type or write a neat copy that he can keep in your records. Sometimes just writing it down will suggest something you could do yourself and you won't need to see him at all – maybe you can buy something without prescription that will do the job.

Take Someone with You
If you're not confident of being able to communicate everything you want to say, take a friend or family member with you. Write the list as above, brief your companion thoroughly in advance and let them do most of the talking for you. This can be especially helpful if you're embarrassed about something.

Ask Him to Write it Down
It's said that a first year medical student learns more new words than someone studying Russian. I'm not sure if it's true, but the profession certainly has its share of distinctive words. If your doctor says you have something you've never heard of, ask him to write the words down. You'll find it difficult to look something up if you don't know how it's spelt! If you tell the doctor you're going to research it, he may write down a few more terms to help you. A good doctor is always happy to help if you're taking an active interest in managing your condition.

Keep Him Informed
Your medical records (in the UK) live with your GP and any specialists you see through the NHS will send necessary updates to them. If you have treatment outside of the NHS (or even in a different county), it's a good idea to tell your GP's practice, so that they have a complete record.

Listen to Him
It takes years of studying before a Doctor takes responsibility for your care and they continue to learn throughout their working life. No-one can be an expert on everything, but they are more knowledgeable than most patients realise. I've heard people complain that their doctor is an idiot – and I've seen campaigns on the internet where people share details on how to "force" your doctor to prescribe a new drug or refer you for experimental

surgery. It's possible that some doctors are idiots, but it's more likely that they have good reason for being cautious. By all means, tell him what you'd like, but *listen* to his advice – and ask him to explain his reasoning. There were doctors who refused to prescribe Thalidomide for morning sickness in the 1950s – can you imagine how grateful their patients are?

Be Prepared to Help Him, Too!

Many GP practices have student doctors studying with them. One group practice I used to attend had a great system of arranging for students to speak to people with chronic conditions. The doctor would draw up outside my house with two or three students in his car. I'd let them in, make a cuppa and the doctor would leave. The students knew I had a chronic condition, but no other details. I just had to answer their questions and explain how MS affected my life. I enjoyed these sessions and I believe the students did, too. It gave them an opportunity to see how "normal" a disabled person is in their own home. The doctors were very grateful, and I like to think I've helped to educate the next generation of medics.

Similar schemes exist, in various forms, all over the country. If you have a little time to spare, I'd recommend telling your GP that you're happy to take part in anything they need patients for.

Be Honest

It's said that everyone lies to their doctors. It's human nature to exaggerate or play down any problems we are experiencing, whether we mean to or not. But we get better advice if we try to be accurate.

A neurologist once told me he'd been asked to diagnose someone with an illness they didn't have. She was applying for asylum in the UK and thought it would help if she had a chronic illness. He'd been scrupulously honest about his findings, both with her and in his report. Although she had tried to fake symptoms, he'd seen through her and refused to co-operate when she came clean and asked him to lie for her.

Your doctor is best placed to help you if he has an accurate picture of your problem. Assuming you're asking for his help, of course. What you tell your employer or the Government is not my concern, but a doctor is likely to see through any faking, whether he says so or not. And I for one would rather have him on my side.

Carrying Information

I carry a piece of paper in my wallet with details of my condition, a list of my usual medication and contact details for my next of kin. It's in the front, with my donor cards and a photo of my husband. If you want to be smart, you can print this on a credit card-sized piece of paper and get it laminated. You may never need it, but it's good to have it handy if you ever do.

Check Your Medication

Shake me – I rattle. Most of the tablets I take first thing in the morning are preventative – fish oils for my joints and calcium for bones. But it's still quite a handful. Many people take a cocktail of prescribed medicines every day – and never stop to question whether they need them all. Some medicines prevent others from working or interact to give unwanted side effects. Sometimes people keep taking medicines they no longer need because no-one questions the prescription. If you get prescriptions from more than one doctor, they may not realise what else you are taking. Whatever the reason, it's worth having a review of your medicines on a regular basis. You could ask your GP to go over everything with you – or your local pharmacist. It doesn't take long and it can be very useful.

Not to mention saving you money if you're paying for a treatment that isn't helping anymore!

Expert Patients Program

There's a scheme in the UK called the Expert Patients Program. It's a really helpful little course designed to teach you how to manage your long-term condition. The idea is to accept that your doctor cannot be an expert in everyone's individual ailments, so you try to become an expert yourself. It's not medical training, but about learning ways to cope. Some of the points I've mentioned above are covered, along with practice at problem-solving for each other. The one I attended was a two-hour session each week for six weeks. There was no charge for the course; I learned a few useful tricks and met some really nice people. Ask your doctor or Citizen's Advice Bureau if there's something similar running locally.

Learn to work Together

Although patients and doctors have their differences, the main thing is to remember that we all want the same thing – our continued health. Even if we approach this aim from different directions, it's possible for both sides of the relationship to benefit from co-operating with each other. A good doctor wants you to be as well as possible. Next time you disagree with a doctor, try to see it from their side and see if you can learn a better way of working together next time.

The Blues

Symptom Poker

The title of this chapter is a phrase I invented as a shorthand for the way some people discuss their illnesses. The conversation goes something like this:

"Hello Meg. You look well. How are you?"

"Fair to middling. Tired all the time, but what's new?"

"Oh, I know exactly what you mean. I'm really tired – and my back hurts."

There are certain people who always do that. Whatever symptom I'm suffering from – they got that worse than me, and at least one other as well. In poker terms:

"I see your fatigue and I raise you a bad back."

Symptoms as a sort of bidding war. To what end? Is she trying to prove she's worse off than I am or just that I'm not really ill? I don't know and honestly don't care. I'll sympathise with anyone who's suffering, but it's much harder when they feel they have to play this game of one-downmanship. I hate this conversational tactic. She's not just saying her own illness is bad, but she's implying that mine is hardly worth mentioning.

The other side of symptom poker is the way some people use a question about someone's health solely as a way to get their own problems into the conversation. I was helping to host an open mic event when someone made a performance of sitting at my table, knocking a chair over and clattering her walking stick onto the floor.

"What's your problem, then?" she asked, gesturing at my crutches, propped against the table.

"I have MS," I reply, shrugging.

"Oh, nothing serious then. I have osteoarthritis – that's much worse."

What can you say? I'm sure it's a difficult condition to live with and she may well be suffering far more than I am. I'd be happy to discuss mobility problems with her, as it's something we have in common. But she's opened the discussion by dismissing my symptoms, so she obviously isn't looking to compare notes or ask my advice. If it's a cry for help, there are many polite ways of opening a discussion. I made my excuses and moved to another table.

Too Tall, Too Short and Possibly Too Fat

For as long as I can remember, I've been taller than most of my peers. I dropped out of ballet lessons when it became obvious I was several inches higher than the standard for ballerinas. So it came as a bit of a shock to find I'm now shorter than the majority of adults– at least when I'm in my wheelchair. There is a lot more to it than just needing help to reach the top shelf in a shop, as I found once I was in this position - so to speak.

The companies that make clothing for wheelchair users never have an "extra long" in the range and their clothes are so boring! Most of my clothes come from shops that specialise in clothing for tall women. It's expensive, but that's life. If I want jeans that come in sight of my ankles, or a dress that curves in the right places, I have to pay a premium. I've thought about having a few items adjusted, so I could have one pair of trousers without bulky, excess fabric in my lap if I'm going to spend all day in a wheelchair. There's a strange sort of irony in having to buy clothing suitable for tall people, but being too short to reach the buttons in a lift!

The observant reader will have noticed I haven't mentioned my actual height yet. There's a good reason for this – it depends how you measure me. One of the consequences of reduced mobility is that you lose height. Medical professionals disagree on the reasons, but the bottom line is that you get shorter if you don't stand or walk much, just as an elderly person does.

So how tall am I? Well, a few years ago, I had my height measured by a very accurate laser device at a science fair. They gave me a certificate which states that I was 1.78m (5' 10" in old money). When I was measured recently by a fitness instructor, she hurried me under the measure and took her reading before I could straighten myself out; she insisted I was only 1.7m (5' 7"). To resolve the issue, I asked my GP's opinion. He measured me carefully, allowing me time to stand up properly. He found me to be 1.76m (5' 9¼"). So I've lost 2cm or a little under an inch in height as a result of restricted mobility.

Does this really matter? Height is just a measurement, after all. True – but don't forget those official guidelines. We're often ridiculously keen to measure and weigh everything against targets. Many medics prefer labelling their patients to spending the time on a fuller picture of a person's health. A UK Government guideline states that women with a waist measurement of more than 88cm (34½") are at increased risk from certain medical problems. (It's 102cm or 40" for men.) The guideline implies that I'm not at risk as long as my waist stays below 88cm – and the same applies to a friend who's only a little taller than me when I'm in my wheelchair and she's standing. Wouldn't it make more sense to quote the target waist measurement as a percentage of a person's height? Interestingly, similar guidelines exist in Japan, derived from the same research by the International Diabetes Federation. But in Japan, they use a slightly larger measurement for women (90cm or 35½") and a *much* smaller one for men (85cm or 33½"). These measurements may be important, but their interpretations are somewhat arbitrary.

The waist measurement problem is further compounded by the natural loss of muscle tone in that area from not standing upright very often. I know a couple of wheelchair users who have been told to lose weight simply because their waist is seen as too big. Some people call this "jelly belly", some have less polite terms for it.

I confess I carry more fat than I'd like to. It's inevitable, given my difficulties in exercising and my love of good food. Yes, I'm sure I could be slimmer if I gave up everything that's bad for me – but I'm not sure I'd be any happier. So I compromise. When I left work in 2004 I was clinically obese. (My BMI[2] fell into the 30~35 bracket). As my health had been so bad for so long, I'd had a lot more to worry about than my weight – and it showed.

Since then, I've been shedding pounds steadily. This isn't a book about dieting, so I won't bore readers with the details (but see chapter *You Shouldn't Eat That* for more comments on diet and MS). Suffice it to say, over the years I have achieved my goal of dropping out of "obese" and into "overweight". This makes a considerable difference with doctors, nurses and so on – crossing that threshold stops them nagging me about my flabby bits. Well, mostly. The fitness instructor who under-measured me, also weighed me (fully clothed in boots, jeans and jumper) and concluded that I was still obese. This short word affected what she was prepared to let me do in the gym as well as feeling she was justified in lecturing me on healthy eating. Instead of her helping me to identify which exercises I could do for maximum benefit, she decided that the important thing was for me to lose weight. I missed out on a potentially helpful resource simply because she inaccurately labelled me as "obese".

---

[2] Body Mass Index. A measure of "fatness". To be technical, it's (weight in kilograms) divided by (height in metres) squared. A value of 20~25 is considered "normal," 25~30 means overweight, 30~35 obese, then morbidly obese and so on. You may hear slightly different values for these thresholds, depending on who you ask, but I've stuck to the simplest ones.

On the whole, I'm a fan of BMI as a measure. It combines height and weight into a single figure, which can then be used as part of a person's physical assessment. Yes, it has its flaws – professional rugby players tend to come up as obese because of their muscle mass, for example. But it's better than most. I believe it's more important to be reasonably fit and healthy than slim, but those are harder to measure, and many professionals take the easy option of looking at BMI alone instead of the wider picture.

So where does this leave us? I would say it's important to apply a little more thought to issues of height, weight etc. Since so many people are hung up on simple measurements, it's worth insisting they give you time to stand up straight when they measure you. Then suggest that they check your blood pressure and resting pulse as a better indication of your general fitness than your BMI alone. Being overweight isn't good for disabled people or anyone else, and I'm not suggesting disability is an excuse for morbid obesity resulting from a poor diet. Too much weight is bound to worsen other physical conditions, but perhaps being fit and happy are more important than getting hung up on reaching your ideal weight.

Daytime TV and Other Terrors

With a variable condition like MS, it's difficult to have a regular daily routine. Yes, I have days when I can write for hours and still have the energy left to cook a meal in the evening. I also have days when I struggle to even sit upright and send my Hubby out for take-away pasta from our local Italian. Which begs the question – what do I do with myself on these fatigue-days?

I have a very real fear of getting sucked into the black hole of daytime TV programmes. I'm sure plenty of people enjoy that mix of soap operas, confession shows, property shows, chat shows... but I'm afraid of disappearing into the schedule and never surfacing again. Radio is better – I like talk stations rather than music during the day. Feels like company...

For the first few months after I left full-time work, I was too ill to do much of anything. I'd dragged myself into the office every day until I literally couldn't get out of bed. Looking back, I can hardly remember anything about that summer. I know I cooked, ate, took phone calls; but the whole period blends into a grey haze. I stayed in bed much of the day, not bothering to dress. I ate whatever snacks were handy. I don't think I'd have had the energy to turn the telly on, even if I'd thought of it!

Then the haze started to clear. I picked up a book and started reading for the first time in months. I put some music on and dug out my neglected knitting. I think the cat was first to notice that I'd woken up – long before I realised. I wasn't well, but I was functioning as a human being again.

Several years later, I know how easy it is for me to slide back into that greyness. If you don't have to go into the office every day, it's tempting to not bother getting dressed. There are take-aways and ready meals, so it's never necessary to actually cook anything. And hey, who needs to clean? I can go a whole week without speaking to a single person except my Hubby. So I have rules. I'm allowed to bend them, even break them occasionally, but I take them seriously enough to feel guilty about skipping one. Every day, I try to write something, exercise, speak to someone, do something crafty (usually knitting) and eat at least one proper meal. Doesn't sound like much, does it? But sometimes even that short list is too much for me. A little more detail:

Write Something. Writing is important to me. I always have at least two projects on the go – usually one factual and one fiction. At the time of writing I'm working on this book (!), a couple of magazine pieces and a radio play. The advantage of having multiple simultaneous works is that I can't use getting "blocked" as an excuse not to write. If I get stuck on one, I switch to another for a while. Some days I don't actually write anything, but I try to get my brain working on plot twists. Or thinking of new chapters for this ever-growing volume!

Exercise. On a good day, I spend a few minutes stretching, lifting weights and then move on to aerobic exercise. It wouldn't look very impressive to an able-bodied person. It would have looked pathetic to me 20 years ago! But it's enough to help keep my poor old body flexible and as mobile as possible. I find it's a great mood-lifter, too – especially when I don't feel like making the effort. Very quickly, I feel much happier with myself, even if I can barely sit up unaided. Disability makes it hard to exercise, but I don't accept it as an excuse not to bother. I honestly believe that without my exercises, I would no longer be able to get out of the wheelchair. Yes it's hard. It can be painful. But it's worth it!

Speak to Someone. If you're stuck at home with a chronic illness, it's easy to see how disabled and elderly people develop agoraphobia. The first time Hubby had to go away on business when I was at home, I welcomed him back at the end of the week – and realised I'd literally not spoken to another human being all week. It's so easy. No-one had rung the doorbell and I hadn't left the house. I couldn't have been more isolated if I'd been on Mars. Since then, I make more of an effort. If I'm on my own, I make a point of leaving the house every day, even if it's just a trip into town for an Americano at my favourite café. This way, I can be sure to interact with other people. Because I travel on my buggy to get there, I usually see someone I know – or meet someone new – and stop for a quick chat. We're a gregarious species and it's good to talk!

Craft Something. I've always got a few projects on the go. When my hands are playing up, I can only knit chunky wool on the thickest of needles, but most of the time I can manage finer work, or tapestry, cross-stitch, fancy leatherwork or something else. I love crafting and get a real kick out of seeing someone wearing a jumper I've made. Knitting is especially good for the soul. I love to sit, listening to an audio book or the radio, knitting something and negotiating with the cat for custody of the wool ball.

Eat a Proper Meal. There have been days when I literally don't have the energy to prepare anything to eat. Sometimes I cook a meal and I'm so wiped out that I can't eat it. But I insist on trying. If I'm too tired, I send Hubby out to get something, or cook easy food. Don't knock fish fingers and oven chips! If Hubby isn't around, I sometimes combine this rule with the one about speaking to someone, by eating a meal at our local pub or our local Italian restaurant, where the welcome is as good for me as the food. It's particularly seductive when I'm on my own to just graze instead of eating real food, but it's a dangerous way to live!

Yes, I do sometimes watch TV during the day. It's more likely to be something I've recorded than actual daytime telly, but I'm still sitting with my face pointed at the goggle-box. I'm likely to be knitting, though. Or eating a hot meal off a tray.

Drunk and Disorderly - or Disabled

"Excuse me, should you be riding that?" He was a Community Support Officer – one I hadn't met before.

"Hello Officer, yes – he's my buggy. I'm always around town on him. You're new here, aren't you?"

"Erm, yes, I've only just joined the force. But you still shouldn't be riding that."

"No, it's fine. I don't drive anymore, so this is how I get around town," I replied. Was he trying to tell me I had to be a pensioner to ride an electric scooter?

"I don't think you should drive after you've been drinking," he said, looking embarrassed.

The penny dropped.

"You think I'm drunk!" I said. "At ten o'clock in the morning?"

"Not at all. I'm just not sure you should be driving."

"Officer, I'm not drunk. I haven't had any alcohol since dinner yesterday. That's not why I can't walk properly, honest!"

Now he really was blushing. I took pity on him.

"Look – I have MS, that's why I walk on crutches. Even then, I can look pretty unsteady, but I'm perfectly safe to ride my little buggy."

"Erm, but..." He gestured towards my face but didn't continue.

"Am I slurring?" I looked him in the eye, ignoring his red face. "That's because of the MS, too. You're welcome to breathalyse me, if you want."

He declined, but I don't think he was convinced.

Like all of our local police officers, he's now used to seeing me ride around town – and the difficulties I have when I stand up. I know he was only doing his duty and I really don't mind the police checking I'm safe to ride. Our local police are a great bunch and very helpful to those of us on wheels.

It's easy to see why someone might think I'm drunk. I have difficulty walking, I sometimes slur my words and I can doze off if I sit quietly for long. Of course, I might do any of those when I've been drinking, too!

It's not so much of a problem when I'm in my wheelchair, as I don't stagger and most people can't tell if I'm finding it difficult to wheel in a straight line. But I know how it appears when I wobble on my crutches. It used to trouble me far more when my disability was less obvious, because of the assumptions people made. It's easier to ignore them now as they can see I'm disabled – and I've grown used to telling people it's none of their business if they make a snide remark.

I often hit problems on the phone, when I realise I'm slurring my words a little and have to apologise to the person I'm speaking to. I get the feeling they don't believe me – but if I'm speaking less than intelligibly at ten o'clock in the morning, I promise you – it's not because of the booze! It amazes me that people employed to speak to customers on the phone can be so rude about a speech impediment – especially when they have such a strong regional accent that many of us would have trouble understanding what they're saying.

There are other aspects of a disability that can be misconstrued. Any form of speech difficulty or hearing problem seems to automatically lead to an assumption that the sufferer is of limited intelligence. Actually, any form of visible disability has that effect, too. See chapter "Does She Take Sugar?" for more ranting on that subject.

Money Matters

It's a well-known fact that all disabled people are completely naive about money. It must be true - I've come across so many people who tell me so. Fortunately, some of us don't believe it and are happy to prove otherwise, but there are certain areas that can be difficult.

Firstly, benefits. Contrary to popular belief and media commentary, disabled people do not automatically qualify for huge handouts from the public purse. The majority of State benefits in the UK are only paid after household income has been confirmed, to ensure the money goes to those who need it most. At the time of writing, the only non-means tested benefit open to most disabled people is Disability Living Allowance, an acknowledgement that having a disability costs money, so the amount paid is based on the severity of the recipient's condition. Help can also be available in the form of free glasses, prescriptions and bus passes. Many people do not claim the benefits they are entitled to, whether through pride or not knowing the ins and outs of the welfare system. I'd advise anyone to consult their local Citizens' Advice Bureau (CAB) for up-to-date information on what they may be able to claim and how to go about it. When asked to explain how your condition affects you, the official advice (which I agree with) is to talk about yourself as you feel on an average day. Don't be noble and insist it isn't a problem, but don't exaggerate, either. Be honest.

Secondly, buying products related directly to your disability. If you're buying something to "enable" yourself, you should be able to buy it without paying VAT. Shops specialising in disability products are used to this and will have a form you sign to say that you're entitled to receive it VAT-free and they handle the paperwork. *But* this rule can also be applied to other purchases – such as new cars. The rules for car purchase are complicated and worth checking in advance. Roughly, the car must be new, bought directly from the dealer and modified *on their premises before purchase* to suit your needs. As long as you need a modification, such as hand controls or a hoist to lift your wheelchair in and out, then you should qualify. In theory, all sorts of purchases could come VAT-free, but in reality you're restricted to those you can buy from retailers who understand the process and are prepared to help. In particular, I've never heard of anyone buying a PC VAT-free, although I know several people who've tried.

So why are we all so naive about money? I based that statement on my experiences of sellers thinking they can charge over-the-top prices for products because they're aimed at the disability market. A disability store regularly short-changes me until I point it out. In the same store, items of chunky-handled cutlery were being sold individually. They would have been helpful for someone with limited dexterity, true – but I noticed a box at the back with a familiar type of stock control tag still attached. I made a note of the number and checked it in the Argos catalogue when I got home. Sure enough, it was the same cutlery – 24 pieces for £13.99. More than a 1,000% mark-up when they were sold individually for £6.49. Be aware and beware – can you buy a similar product elsewhere without paying a premium for the "disability" tag?

The worst example I encountered personally was in looking for a new wheelchair, five years ago. I'd decided which model I wanted, the frame colour, correct seat size and everything. All the options I wanted were available automatically from the manufacturer – no additional charge involved. So I went to three local retailers for quotes. All of them told me I'd have to pay extra for at least one of the options and / or delivery. Two of them tried very hard to sell me additional products from their shop. The lowest price I was quoted was equal to the Recommended Retail Price – but delivery was extra and he told me I couldn't have the colour I wanted.

I looked on the internet, sent a couple of emails and bought the exact tailor-made one I wanted, for 20% less than the RRP, colour, size and delivery included. It pays to shop around.

As I write this chapter, I've repeated the same exercise, with a current wheelchair model, including a few options that the manufacturers include in the basic price. I used my favourite search engine to look for *wheelchair <model-name> UK* and found three retailers offering it for less than the RRP. The shops I phoned all quoted considerably more and told me the "extras" would involve additional charges. Nothing has changed.

With such differences in prices charged, it's well worth the time it takes to check out available prices. The internet is our most potent weapon in this war, even if it means enlisting the help of a tech-savvy friend (or helpful librarian) to do some of the work for you. As long as some retailers assume we'll pay what they ask because we don't know any better, we need to be alert and seek out the ones who reward our ability to find them. There *are* shops which don't charge extra for things that are included in the basic price, so it's not just the need to cover their overheads. You could save £100s on a wheelchair, £1,000s on a new car – simply by checking what's available.

I'm not accusing all shops specialising in disability equipment of ripping us off, but it's important to be wary. Remember, they aren't charities – they're in business to make money and we don't have to be as naive as some of them think we are.

Paranoia

par·a·noi·a [par-uh-noi-uh]
—noun   1. Psychiatry. a mental disorder characterized by systematized delusions and the projection of personal conflicts, which are ascribed to the supposed hostility of others, sometimes progressing to disturbances of consciousness and aggressive acts believed to be performed in self-defence or as a mission. 2. baseless or excessive suspicion of the motives of others.

Like many mental disorders, paranoia is often seen as a bit of a joke. There is a whole spectrum of paranoia – from normal, human fears that people are laughing at our choice of clothes to life-dominating fears about worldwide conspiracies. The shade I want to address lies somewhere between these – it's the possibly-correct suspicion that people are picking on you because of your disability.

There can be no doubt that we are perceived as being different by virtue of our disability. There aren't enough people around in wheelchairs for the sight to be taken for granted. Of course, not everyone who reacts to a visible disability does so in a negative way – or intentionally negative, anyway.

Some years ago, a campaign was launched by a disability charity, using the slogan, "See the Person, not the Wheelchair". They used a picture of an attractive young woman sitting in a wheelchair. Stark naked. An effective way to get a point across! She was posed very demurely, fig-leafed by her arm and leg – but very obviously not wearing any clothes. I defy anyone to view that picture and see the wheelchair first!

But, in the real world, the wheelchair *is* the first thing people see. Or the white stick, crutches, guide dog or whatever. Since we can't use nudity as a distraction tactic in our everyday lives, we have to accept that the disability is going to be the first thing most people notice about us.

Is this a bad thing, though? Surely most people will react positively to our evident problems and therefore we will get the help we need, without having to make a fuss about it.

And I've got this Gloucester Old Spot with lovely markings on his wings.

Some people do react positively to evident disabilities. Many think they're reacting well, but actually make things worse. A certain type of person likes to be seen to help – but doesn't really do anything to make our lives easier. A large percentage of the population try not to see the person at all. And there *are* those who see any disabled person as a target.

Or am I being paranoid?

I have come across people in each of these categories and plenty of variations in between. I've also been accused of being paranoid – usually by someone who's trying to manoeuvre me into doing something for them at my own cost. Maybe I am a little paranoid, but maybe I'm only seeing what's really going on.

There's no denying it's hard to distinguish between paranoia and being picked on, it's often little more than a matter of perspective. A recent conversation:

"So how's Meg?" asked the woman behind the counter.

"Ticking over, you know," I replied.

"Oh, do your legs hurt?"

"Don't ask," I said, shaking my head.

"Ok, I won't. Is it very bad?"

"Don't ask."

"It must be terrible for you. You know I'm here if you ever want to talk to someone. Do your legs hurt a lot of the time?"

I walked away. I know it's rude of me, but it's the politest way I could think of to end the conversation. She waited until I was settled with my coffee and sat down opposite.

"Do you often get days when it hurts this much?"

I sighed. "I said *don't ask* – what did you think I meant?"

"It must be awful, I know just what it's like to be noble about your suffering. Why's it suddenly hurting you so much?"

"DON'T ASK!" This time I said it loud enough for the manager to hear, before getting up, leaving money for my unfinished coffee and exiting.

When I still worked in an office, I was often told I was being paranoid by other members of staff. At first, I took this at face value, blaming myself for seeing discrimination where it didn't exist and assuming I was being singled out for different treatment. It's only now, several years after leaving the job that I can see just how much discrimination there was. Yes, I was being paranoid some of the time and I'll happily admit some of it was my own fault. But that paranoia grew from a culture of constant anti-disability discrimination.

Disability Charities

When asked for a reliable source of information on any chronic condition, I recommend a charity that supports people with that condition. Most charities are very helpful at providing booklets or making info available on their website. Many fund specific services– such as specialist nurses, drop-in centres, respite care, etc. I've given a lot of time and money to various charities over the years and will continue to do so.

The observant reader will have noticed on the cover of this book that I promise to make a 50p payment to MS charities for every copy I sell. I don't specify which charities for a very good reason: I reserve the right to change the beneficiary without notice. Charities do a lot of good work - raising money, funding research, publicising disability, providing services that would otherwise not be available. I've had excellent support, advice and information from them over the years.

I've also seen bickering inside and between charities; discrimination from people who represent charitable bodies and appalling greed. Charities who assume that having your details on their database means they can bombard you with demands for contributions and "volunteer" work. I understand very well the reasons for people (including celebrities) supporting certain charities and why they sometimes withdraw that support. Charities are big businesses, celebrity endorsements are an essential part of their arsenal, but there are always politics and disagreements behind the scenes, too.

Whilst writing this book, I have approached various groups for assistance. Depending on who I was contacting, I have asked for publicity, endorsements, partnerships and/or financial support (I pay to publish, even though I have always sold enough books to cover costs). I have to admit, I've been disappointed in the responses.

A London-based charity told me they weren't allowed to support me because they're UK-registered and they can't support anything in another country – like Wales. (Which, as the reader probably knows, *is* part of the UK.)

Another charity said they'd consider giving me a quote for the cover, but they needed a bound copy of the book for a couple of months to read before they could comment, and that they'd want a prime position on the cover if they did give me anything. So I'd have to pay for pre-publication and the subsequent changes to the book. And delay publication whilst they read it, all with no guarantee that they'd let me quote them.

One charity thanked me for sending a couple of chapters, saying they would use them immediately and when was I giving them the rest? I pointed out that my email specified the chapters were in draft and not for publication. Especially not without my agreement.

I phoned one charity to ask if they'd support me in any way and received a flat refusal to even discuss my request. A manager at the same charity later told me none of their staff would have dismissed me in this way. I asked what response they should have made and didn't get an answer.

Another body said they'd publish me – electronically. They really liked my work and would be happy to give it away under their own name.

I'm not naming either people or charities in this chapter because it's not my intention to make any sort of trouble and I know this is a litigious culture where I could easily find myself in court for defamation. Some of the above comments can be proven as they were in emails, but

I can't prove what's been said to me over the phone. The idea is to express a general opinion based on my experiences – bad as well as good.

Now, I appreciate that charities have to be careful how they spend the money they've raised and that this little book may not sound useful enough to attract funding. But isn't it worth proper consideration? If my work is good and interesting enough that they'd happily distribute it and take credit– why won't they consider doing something in return?

So this book has been produced with my own money and I will make that contribution to an MS charity when I sell copies. But I'm keeping my options open as to which one it is at any given time.

Accidents and Emergencies
Warning: contains graphic scenes of stupidity, blood and bruises.

I guess they're mostly self-inflicted, but I've had more than my share of accidents, some of which have needed hospital attention. I could have avoided many of them if I'd been more cautious, but I prefer the occasional risk to life in a bubble of my own making.

One of the biggest hazards in my day-to-day life must be the stairs. Yes, I live in a house with stairs and have to go up and down them several times a day. It's getting increasingly difficult, but I prefer to struggle as long as I can. If I'd been sensible and moved into a bungalow some years ago, I reckon I wouldn't be able to manage them at all by now. We've got very sturdy rails on both sides that help a lot. On a bad day, when my legs won't co-operate enough to manage even with the help of the banisters, I sit on the stairs and pull myself up with my arms. Coming down is even less elegant, but it works.

The problem is, even when I think I can manage the stairs, I'm likely to slip. This usually involves nothing more than my foot sliding onto the step below the one I was aiming for, but every now and then I actually fall and collect bruises for a few steps, until I can apply the brakes by bracing my hands against the walls. To date, I've never injured myself beyond some colourful bruises, but I guess it's only a matter of time.

One day, I accidentally kicked the corner of a chest of drawers with my bare foot. I do this kind of thing fairly often, so all I did was swear and carry on where I was going. It took me a few minutes to notice the blood.

In kicking the corner, my little toe had been forced out at right-angles to the next toe, splitting the skin between the two. I didn't feel the damage, only the shock of striking the furniture. I was lucky not to break any bones! Dressing the wound was an interesting exercise in first aid techniques, but it healed just fine and there's only a scar there now.

One of my more spectacular injuries happened when I was cutting bread for our lunch. I held the loaf with my left hand and my reduced sensation failed to inform me that the bread knife had sliced off more than just bread. I had, in fact, cut a diagonal piece off the end of my middle finger. As soon as I realised, I shoved my finger under cold running water and called my Hubby to bring the first aid kit. I tried to stick a plaster over the wound, but couldn't stop the bleeding. I wrapped kitchen roll round the finger, applying pressure to stem the flow – but the blood seeped through. Acknowledging defeat, I told him to get the car and wrapped more kitchen roll round the steadily-growing red and white mass on my hand.

Arriving at our local Accident and Emergency Department, I told the receptionist that I'd cut the end off my finger and couldn't get it to stop bleeding. She looked unimpressed (reasonably enough) and told me to wait until I was called by the triage nurse. I saw more urgent cases being treated as they arrived and sent Hubby home, rather than waste his Saturday afternoon. I waited my turn, adding kitchen roll to the now-huge lump around my hand. Fortunately things were reasonably quiet, so I only had to wait another half an hour before being called.

"Your notes say you've cut your finger," said the triage nurse.

"Well, actually I've cut the end off my finger and I can't stop the bleeding," I replied.

"Why didn't you just put a plaster on it?" she asked.

"I tried, but there's too much blood. I think I've cut an artery."

She gave me a look that nurses have to practice for years. I knew she thought I was making a fuss about nothing, but there was no way for me to convince her I knew what I was talking about. I'd been a qualified first aider before she was born, but there didn't seem much point in mentioning that fact.

"Let's have a look at it," she said as she whipped the kitchen roll away.

My finger spurted a jet of blood in a neat dotted line, right down the front of her uniform.

After that, the staff took my injury a little more seriously. They soon had me lying on a bed, with my wrist tied to an IV stand. They filled a couple of surgical gloves with ice and bandaged these to my hand, all in an attempt to stop the bleeding. They discussed the possibility of stitching it, but that meant removing the rest of my finger nail and would only have made things worse. It took another two hours to persuade the artery to stop spurting blood, at which point the nurses applied several layers of dressing and sent me home with strict instructions not to remove anything from the wound for at least three days and to come straight back if the blood came through again.

Once they'd finished with me, I called Hubby to come and pick me up. He did so and on the way home he told me he'd decided to finish making our interrupted lunch. When he picked up the bread knife, he'd found a little piece of finger with nail still attached. He decided to use a different knife.

Looking back, this has become little more than a funny anecdote, but it taught me an important lesson. Even a small injury can have major implications if it's not dealt with properly. It's common for injuries to MSers to behave oddly, the damaged nerves affecting the normal processes that should halt the bleeding – but I didn't learn that until years afterwards. And I'm fairly sure the nurses didn't know it, either.

I suspect that my arriving in a wheelchair made them more sceptical of my self-diagnosis than they would have been if I'd walked in like anyone else, but I can't be sure. Maybe any patient with a minor arterial bleed would have been left waiting as I was. But if I'm ever there with something life-threatening, I'll make sure they don't push me to the back of the queue.

My Friend Indigo

Trampering

My spellchecker reckons that title isn't a real word. I disagree and I'm bigger than the laptop, so I win.

I am a Tramper owner and this chapter is going to sound like an advert. If you want to know more, visit: http://tramper.co.uk/ for details.

When I mention that I have an electric buggy, I can almost see the image hovering in front of your mind's eye. But that "granny scooter" isn't quite the whole story. Imagine that the scooter you're thinking of has mated with a quad bike and picture their offspring. Now you're getting close. If your picture looks anything like the one on the front cover, then you've got the idea. Legally, he's a Class III mobility vehicle, subject to all the appropriate regulations. But he's a true off-roader and it shows; big, rugged tyres, excellent suspension, proper headlights and the pulling power of a small horse. Oh, and he's purple.

Having a good buggy gives me far more mobility than a traditional mobility scooter would. I live in a very three-dimensional part of the country – the river Severn has carved its way to the sea only a stone's throw away. Being on a Tramper allows me to get around on all these hilly roads, with my crutches or wheelchair on the back. And if we're on holiday, the buggy sits on his own trailer to go with us. I may not be able to walk very far and I'll never drive again – but I do have more mobility than most people in my position.

Not surprisingly, there's no chance of getting such a vehicle provided by the NHS or any other official body. The only way for me to get this useful buggy was to pay for it myself and they aren't cheap! So I budget for my Tramper as if it's the second car that most households run. Suddenly it doesn't look so expensive. Road tax is free for mobility vehicles (although they still have to be registered) and the insurance isn't too bad. He charges from an electrical socket – and from gravity when I'm going downhill. I've ridden him through rain, puddles, mud, sand, snow and gravel.

You'll notice I refer to my buggy as "him". Yes, he has a name and yes, I do talk to him. Just as many people do with their cars.

Having an off-road buggy has made it possible for me to join in with many activities I would be excluded from without him:

- I ride him into town, so I'm not reliant on anyone else to run errands for me.
- I used to ride him into work – including night shifts, so I was riding home at three o'clock in the morning, much to the confusion of our local foxes.
- I've taken him to those holiday villages where cars are banned most of the week and everyone is meant to ride bikes. I particularly enjoy the jealous comments I get from people struggling to pedal uphill!

Advertising aside, these electric scooters can make a tremendous difference to people with limited mobility. I choose to have a buggy with off-road capabilities, as that suits my lifestyle. Some people prefer a lightweight one that folds into the boot of their car. If you're looking for one, decide what you want it to do before you buy – it's a very expensive mistake to choose the wrong one. And worth every penny when you get the right one.

Prince Philip's Steps

Many people have a list of places they'll get round to visiting and most of us never actually do it. There are so many reasons we can't do it this year – it's too expensive; we've got family commitments; I can't get the time off work; who'd look after the cat? Maybe next year.

And maybe next year you won't be well enough.

Ever since I found out my weird symptoms were caused by MS, I've been acutely aware of my failing health. Even if things get a little better for a while, my mobility and other problems have been worsening steadily for years. So "next year" isn't something I can take for granted.

So, I promised myself I'd "get round" to some of that list. Some of these are mentioned in chapter, "Life's Too Short", but the most important one is a dream I've had since I saw David Attenborough present a programme from the Galapagos Islands, more than 30 years ago. These isolated equatorial volcanic islands are so remote the wildlife hasn't learnt to fear humans. Here, Charles Darwin conceived his theory of evolution, observing the way finches and mockingbirds had evolved to eat whatever food supply was available on each island. The exotic animals fascinated me, and the idea of a place where wild creatures didn't fear people was unbelievably attractive to an animal-mad young girl.

We booked a trip to the islands, saved the money (it wasn't cheap!) and I was off to the Galapagos at last!

We stayed on a ship touring between islands and I managed to do everything except for some of the harder walks. Getting into the landing craft was difficult, but I could manage with a little assistance (it's surprising how much upper-body strength you get from walking with crutches). The trip was extraordinary. After decades of dreaming about these incredible islands, I'd expected to be disappointed in the reality; but the islands were even more magical than I'd anticipated.

Galapagos Nature Reserve rules insist you stick to marked paths, and not touch any animals. Unfortunately, no-one has explained this to the animals, so we would be confronted by a footpath filled with iguanas warming themselves in the morning sunshine, unconcerned at people stepping between them. Some of the animals were almost too friendly - sea-lion pups in particular had a habit of coming up to me, looking up with those beautiful, cuddle-me eyes.

We saw Darwin's finches, frigate birds, sharks, turtles, stingrays, giant tortoises, mockingbirds, a sea alive with hundreds of dolphins and much more. But there was one type of bird we hadn't seen. The Galapagos have three species of boobies – seabirds the size of a gannet. (Their name comes from *bobo*, the Spanish word for "clown".) We'd seen blue-footed and masked boobies – but no red-footed boobies. The best way to see these rare creatures is to visit their breeding colony on Genovesa Island, where the web-footed clowns perch with their feet wrapped around branches! Towards the end of our holiday, the boat was moored inside the extinct volcano which forms the island, so we could visit the red-foots.

The Guides had warned that we would have to climb a "staircase" in the caldera wall to get onto the island, but their English (and my Spanish) didn't stretch to a full explanation. It's called *Prince Philip's Steps,* since that gentleman climbed them in 1964. The Queen had declined, and I could see why. From our boat, the steps looked very steep, roughly carved from the volcano's wall; uneven and far too narrow to allow anyone to assist me. I climbed them on my hands and knees, pulling myself up by the handrails in some places. It cost me some bruises and scrapes, but it was worth it. At the top, we walked around trees full of red-foot nests, with these comical birds staring back at us only a few feet away.

After returning to mainland Ecuador, we had arranged to spend a few nights in a "jungle hotel" – a collection of wooden lodges in the rainforest. I'll never complain about the British climate again, having seen how rain can come down in the tropics.

Fortunately it didn't rain much and we were taken on a guided walk through the rainforest proper. All right, it was a fairly tame bit with a clear path, but our guide did coax a wild tarantula out of her burrow to show us. At the start of the walk, he handed out sticks to all of the tourists, except me. He eyed my crutches with suspicion but there was no way I could explain how capable I am on them - and I wasn't even certain I would be able to follow his track. He set off up a very steep slope, adjacent to what I suspect was the usual path. He may have been trying to persuade the foolish disabled foreigner to quit while she could; I don't know. I followed him as best I could and reached the top, aware that he was watching me. I looked up to meet his eyes; he held my gaze and nodded deliberately. Who needs a language in common? The rest of the walk was over much less demanding terrain and I managed with far less effort than several other people.

The Galapagos Islands are incredible. It's a corner of the world where mankind hasn't wiped out half the wildlife and scared the rest into hiding whenever they hear a human footstep. I thought I'd never be able to go there, but I have and I've seen many of the unique species that inhabit this little group of volcanic rocks in the Pacific Ocean. My MonSter didn't stop me living that particular dream.

Coping Strategies

You've only got three choices in life – Give in, Give up or Give it all you've got.

So you've got a chronic illness – or it's someone you love, a friend or a colleague. Whoever it is and whatever the condition, you all need to come to terms with the changes in your lives.

There is no simple one-size-fits-all strategy for coping with anything of this magnitude. Some people prefer to push the problem to the back of their minds while others face it head-on. Some are optimistic about the future, others focus more on the negative aspects of their condition. As with anything else, we each react in our way. One sure thing is that people around you will trot out platitudes when they hear the news. So listen to them – this is one occasion when you might just find a nugget of truth in a cliché. Think carefully about each of these:

"It could be worse." Yes, it could. There are people who'd envy you, however bad your situation feels.

"Count your blessings." Whether you're religious or not, there's always something to be grateful for. Spend time identifying the good things in your life. Supportive friends, loving family members, an opportunity that wouldn't have happened if you were still working. Write a list and add to it when something occurs to you.

"Keep smiling." Better advice than you might think. Science has proved that even faking a smile makes us feel better. Pin a grin on your face, especially when you don't feel like it – you'll be surprised how much it can help.

"At least you know what's wrong." For many of us, uncertainty is the worst thing to live with – even the worst diagnosis is better than not knowing! I had weird symptoms for years and was relieved to finally be told it was MS – I had imagined far worse scenarios.

"What doesn't kill us makes us stronger." Yes, it does. And a long-term health problem puts everything else into perspective.

I've known people write the things that make them happy on little sticky notes and post them around their home. I like to stash things that remind me of good days or people who bring a smile to my face. So in my bill-pile I'll come across a letter from a magazine that's published a piece of my work – something I would never have achieved if I were still working full-time. In my pencil case is an engraved pen from another MSer – a thank-you for counselling him through a bad relapse. I file copies of photos in strange places on my PC, so I come across them when I'm working – good friends I've met through disability-related activities; wonderful places I'd never have visited without the spur of MS. If I tried to ignore the realities of my life, I'd cut myself off from these happy thoughts.

My favourite coping strategy is commonly known as **DABDA** or the five stages of grief. Invented by Elisabeth Kübler-Ross in 1969, it describes five phases of dealing with a major change in circumstances: Denial, Anger, Bargaining, Depression, and Acceptance.

Denial: "This can't be happening to me!"
We go through life hearing about tragedies happening to other people and it comes as a shock when the lightning strikes close to home. In a culture where people expect doctors to be able to cure anything with a pill or a quick op, it's hard to accept that they can't. With an illness that progresses rapidly, the human mind flinches from the reality, wants to push it away, to ignore the situation.

Anger: "I'm going to sue someone!"
A very human reaction. It can be a tremendous boost to vent your spleen, whether you shout at someone else or have a good scream in private. Don't hurt anyone, though – including yourself! Anger is a primitive emotion and it's in our nature for a very good reason – it allows us to exorcise the negatives of our situation and move on. Sorry to sound like an aging hippy, but it's true.

Bargaining: "If I go to church every Sunday, I'll be well again." "If I stop smoking the cancer'll go away."
It's only natural to hope fate / God / the universe can be bargained with – although it rarely works. But many conditions *can* be improved by changing the way you live. Anyone who has limited energy knows the kind of deal they make with their condition: "If I want to go out tonight, I need to take things easy all day." It's up to you who or what you negotiate with and I wish you success in your haggling.

Depression: "What's the point of anything?"
Even without a chronic illness, everyone has their "down days". It's human, it's natural and it's lousy (I could have typed something much stronger, but you get the idea). If it's more than you can cope with, tell someone – a friend with broad shoulders, a doctor, your local vicar, a charity's listening line or even a pet. And tell yourself tomorrow will be better.

Acceptance: "I have MS, but MS doesn't have me." "So these are the cards I've been dealt? On with the game."
If life gives you lemons, make lemonade. If life gives you limes, find someone who's got salt and tequila...

Not everyone goes through all the stages in order, or at all. In my experience, it's common to hop backwards and forwards through the list. Even reaching *Acceptance* is no guarantee that you won't slip into *Depression* or *Anger* for a while. And there aren't any clear divisions between the different states of mind. They're just convenient labels to help you understand what's happening inside you.

There is a danger that people don't progress through the stages. *Denial* and *Anger* can be destructive states of mind, but many people with chronic conditions seem to stick in one or the other for a very long time. It's a particular problem with MS, because it usually strikes in the prime of life and it's hard to accept you have something that cannot be cured. I've seen so many newly-diagnosed MSers chasing the latest treatment or miracle cure, firmly believing that their MonSter *will* be destroyed because it can't happen to them. By refusing to acknowledge the need to *Bargain* – to adapt to their changed circumstances and learn to live with it - they leave themselves vulnerable to the worst type of *Depression* and its impact. *Bargaining* and *Acceptance* aren't about giving up on the search for a cure, just making life more bearable in the meantime.

Because of the way I found out that I had MS, I went through *Denial* very quickly – I was so relieved to finally know what was causing all those weird symptoms, I didn't even consider wishing it away. My *Anger* was largely directed at the medical profession who'd concealed my diagnosis for years - but it never took any concrete form. *Bargaining* is something I still do every time I bully myself into exercising when I'd rather rest - I keep my MonSter at bay by constantly fighting him. Yes, I have my spells of *Depression*, days when I'm so weepy I simply avoid everyone else and wait for my mood to lift. I like to think I spend most of my life in a form of *Acceptance*. Except when I don't!

For me, the importance of this model is that it justifies my feelings. It's hard enough to cope with a disability and the moods it causes, without feeling guilty about them. If I'm angry about having to live with a MonSter, I tell myself I'm allowed to rant and scream. And if anyone tells me different, that's their problem – not mine. I've had people say I shouldn't be miserable or angry – but I know that my feelings are natural and it's wrong to tell me otherwise. If you won't give me space to live with my MonSter, please don't expect me to make space for you.

When I tried to explain my emotional situation to a doctor, I described myself as balancing on a point between depression, fear, pride and acceptance. For anyone who knows how poor a sense of balance I have, it's an amusing picture, so perhaps I should describe myself as *wobbling* on that point. That word pride is an important one. Our culture sees pride as a negative emotion and we rarely admit to feeling it. But what other term can I use to explain why I try so hard to hide my disability? I met with a friend recently in a café, wearing a heavy jumper to conceal the colourful bruises on my arms and collar bones; I wouldn't look at him because it would have been obvious that my eyes were misbehaving. Why did I do it? He knows about my falling and my eyesight, so why hide the evidence? David's not easily fazed, but I find myself trying to protect everyone else from my MonSter. I find I wobble a lot towards the pride side. Too much may be a bad thing, but I want to maintain the appearance of normality, or as good an approximation as I can manage. Pride is an important part of my own coping strategy.

I've also been accused of being a control freak. Like pride, wanting to be in control is seen as a bad thing – but is it really so wrong? My MonSter has robbed me of control in many aspects of my life, can you begrudge me the little I have left?

There are as many coping strategies as there are people. I believe the important thing is to recognise the need to cope, rather than ignore the realities; but you're welcome to disagree if you have a system that works better for you.

Life's Too Short

One of the few advantages of a chronic, progressive illness is the way it focuses your mind on your own mortality. I know how strange that sounds, but it's a truth some of us have come to acknowledge.

It may be an uncomfortable subject, but none of us lives forever and it's difficult to ignore the issue when disability brings it into sharp focus every day.

Back in my pre-MS days, I was as happy as anyone to put things off until some remote time in the future, when I would have more time / money / opportunity to do them. I never made firm plans - I just assumed I'd do everything when I retired. Or sometime.

Then, suddenly, I had a disability to cope with.

When coming to terms with the impact of my condition, I did some serious soul-searching about my priorities in life and adjusted them accordingly. It's not an easy thing to do, but I'm glad I took the time. Learning that you're unlikely to have the long, healthy life you'd always assumed you were entitled to, makes you start to re-think your plans. I had to retire from full-time work fifteen years earlier than we'd planned. Our household's income dropped and we started to rethink many things we'd taken for granted.

Everyone has a few places they've always wanted to see and we decided it was worth visiting at least some of mine whilst I was still able to appreciate them properly. So, in the years since I accepted that MS was here to stay:

I have climbed to the mouth of Mount Vesuvius. It's a difficult, dusty climb from the coach park, even outside of the hot season and it's incredibly hard to breathe when you're going uphill with your weight forward on a pair of crutches. But I did it. Please don't ask me to do it again.

I have ridden in a small inflatable boat on a Norwegian fjord in January, watching black fins slicing through the water while herring jump out to escape the herding orcas.

I have stood on the Great Wall of China. Happily, we visited this incredible country before the 2008 Olympics accelerated the westernisation of their ancient culture. We visited siheyuans and hutongs which were later demolished for the Bird's Nest stadium and mounted the Wall to see it snaking across the hills in both directions. We saw the excavation of the Terracotta army near Xi'an. Accessibility was a major issue, especially away from the tourist attractions, but people were friendly and willing to help the idiot westerner who misjudged a kerb and toppled her wheelchair into the street.

I have crossed the equator at the Galapagos Islands. This has been my dream holiday destination for decades and there's more about this in chapter "Prince Philip's Steps".

So, despite my disability, I've seen some of the world's most wonderful sights. In fact, because of my disability. Let's face it – I would still have been putting everything off if I didn't have MS to spur me into making the most of my life! There are still many places I would like to visit, but accessible destinations are less urgent. I hope to see Canada, New Zealand and Japan. There are animal habitats I would dearly love to experience and scenery I hope to be overwhelmed by.

Also as a direct result of having a chronic illness, I learnt to shoot a recurve bow (reaching "First Class

Archer" status); although if I were to continue with that, I'd have to shoot in a disabled category as I'd now need to use some of the aids permitted for those who can't shoot without them. I've joined groups that I wouldn't have had time for if I was still working. See section *The Rainbow and Other Happy Places* for more detail on some of these. I'm active on several sites on the internet – mainly writing and disability ones. And I'm writing – something I hadn't had time for since school.

A disabled friend told me he'd been given six months to live. After the initial shock, he spent his days putting things in order – contacting people he hadn't spoken to in years and suchlike. He found it strangely comfortable to know what was happening. Five years later, the doctors admitted they might have made a mistake about his condition. But he's pleased he had the "kick" that made him focus on what was really important to him.

There is always a silver lining, however dark the cloud.

Two Kinds of Youth

Warning: contains mild offensive and anti-disability language.

Some years ago, riding my buggy home from work one afternoon, I approached a parade of shops I needed to pass. A group of young people in hoodies were hanging around outside. One of them spotted me and I heard him call out,

"Oi, spazz-mobile!"

His friends joined in.

"Hey, missus. My mate fancies you!"

"Can I ave your spazz-mobile, Spastic?"

Once they'd run out of witty remarks (I haven't recorded their nastier ones here), they just chanted,

"Spastic, spazz-mobile, spastic, spazz-mobile..."

I kept my eyes on the road ahead, not wanting to encourage them any further and hoping they couldn't see my tears. I knew I couldn't get away if they decided to chase and that my buggy could be badly damaged - as could I. Thankfully, they limited themselves to abuse and didn't move away from the shop wall they were propping up.

Out of sight of the shops, I found myself trembling. I didn't dare stop in case they followed me, so just continued towards home. About a quarter of a mile further on, I realised I was about to overtake another couple of youths in hoodies, dawdling along the pavement in front of me. I actually considered turning round and taking a different route home, but it would have meant a ridiculous detour, and having to pass close to the shops. I chose to keep on and hoped they wouldn't react as badly as the first group.

The shorter of the boys must have heard my electric motor, and he turned to look. Then he grabbed his friend's sleeve and the two of them stood to one side, giving me plenty of room to pass them. They smiled at me, greeting my buggy with,

"Wow – cool!"

"Wicked!!!!"

I tried to smile back, probably not very successfully. Then one of them called,

"Gis a lift up the hill?"

I stopped. The shorter one was smiling and I noticed he was carrying one of his trainers. Hence the slow walking pace. I told him how to hang on the back and took him to the top of the hill, where he thanked me profusely.

It's not just hoodies who've surprised me over the years. I've met Goths who want to chat about disability and uniformed policemen who literally wouldn't give me the time of day. Obviously, I shouldn't judge able-bodied people by their appearance, tempting though it is. Many of them can be friendly, even when I don't expect it.

Dear Winner

Congratulations, YOU are the lucky winner of a multiple sclerosis prize! YOUR body passed the qualifying rounds and won the final selection!! There is no need to sign for delivery.

You may be wondering how YOU were chosen to win this life-changing prize. In accordance with all legal systems and local by-laws, the final draw is entirely random; although we consider several criteria in the early stages of the selection process. These include gender (we pick 50% more women than men), age, ethnicity, childhood infections, your home region and any close relatives who may have been lucky enough to win previously. Prizes are usually presented between the ages of 25 and 45, although in exceptional cases it may arrive earlier or later.

As the happy recipient of this award, we understand you're impatient to learn more. You'll notice little change in your body's appearance and behaviour at first; but will soon see our gift's growing influence. What begins as a little numbness today may become chronic pain, localised loss of sensation or vicious pins and needles tomorrow. Who knows? In twenty years' time, you may be completely unable to walk. Or you may appear perfectly well. One of the great joys of playing host to multiple sclerosis is never knowing what it will surprise you with next!

Initially, YOUR award will be classed as the relapsing-remitting type. With this diagnosis, you will receive new delights on an irregular basis. YOUR multiple sclerosis will amaze you with its ability to invent original symptoms on its own unpredictable timetable. Any day now, you could be unable to speak clearly or walk in a straight line. Hours of amusement as you try to convince police officers you're not drunk and disorderly!

You've probably noticed some of the basic functions of your prize already. That wobbling of your eyes is called "Nystagmus". We gave it a really obscure name so that no-one will understand what you're complaining about. It's sometimes called "Optic Neuritis" – which is almost as good. That weird way your foot flops about when you're trying to walk? We call that "Drop Foot". A nice, easy term to remember, but it means nothing to anyone else, so you still won't be troubled by any embarrassing sympathy.

Although we don't provide a manual with your prize, you will soon learn the correct terminology for its advanced features. The painful band around your chest that stops you breathing is known as the "MS Hug". They're an ironic bunch in our marketing department. And that sudden feeling of being too tired to even sit up? That's called "MS Fatigue". If you mention it to anyone, they'll assume you're just feeling a bit tired and making a big fuss about nothing.

There are many benefits of ownership you won't notice at first. Your employer will want to discuss your sudden eligibility for early retirement. Non-prize-winning friends will respond to your changing situation – not returning phone calls, forgetting to invite you on a night out, crossing the street when they see you. Don't worry; they're only jealous. You'll make new friends when you start to meet other prize-winners. After all, who understands you better than another lucky recipient?

For obvious commercial reasons, we cannot disclose the long-term behaviour of your award. We do, however, refer you to the countless lies, scare stories, conspiracy theories and quack remedies currently circulating on the internet. One of these may even be a cure, or maybe it's the placebo effect. We aren't saying! Many happy hours can be wasted in a quest to understand the MonSter. Remember, this award has been uniquely designed for YOU and is non-transferable.

Welcome to the fastest-growing community of neurological prize-winners in the world. Welcome to a future with your new, closest companion: a MonSter that will remain with you for the rest of your life.

Yours insincerely,
The Multiple Sclerosis MonSter

To Whom it May Concern

To Whom it May Concern,
As you are probably aware, the writer of this letter has a condition called Multiple Sclerosis – MS for short. Many aspects of this illness are not widely understood and I'd like to take a few minutes of your time to explain some of the commonest problems.

First of all, MS is unpredictable. Most MSers have what's called *relapsing-remitting MS*, which means it gets worse (a relapse) and better (a remission) at unpredictable intervals. However, some have *progressive* forms of the illness and a lucky few have what is known as *benign MS*. Unfortunately for the person concerned, being diagnosed with one type doesn't make their condition predictable and it may change its behaviour without notice. Simply put – MS does what it wants, when it wants and there's nothing anyone can do about it. That's one reason we call it the MonSter.

Some symptoms of MS are obvious –walking sticks and wheelchairs are easy to spot, the strange way of walking and slurred speech too. But the worst facets of this illness are usually invisible. Fatigue is commonly cited as the most debilitating symptom – not just feeling a bit tired, but your energy suddenly draining away, leaving you unable to sit upright or hold a conversation.

MS can affect every part of the body. From icy hands that can't hold a cup without spilling it to eyes that dance around when you're trying to focus on something; from difficulty in swallowing to weakness and muscle spasms that leave you unable to walk; from bladder, bowel and digestive problems to cognition and memory difficulties. Nothing is safe from the MonSter and nothing is sacred.

"But they've cured MS, haven't they? All those wonderful new drugs!" No, there is no cure. There are treatments that reduce the severity of MS in some cases, but they're expensive, can be hard to get hold of and they don't work for everyone. The long-term prognosis for anyone with MS is not good. Their level of disability steadily worsens over time, but this can take decades and many MSers live long, productive lives. Meanwhile, the media love to report miracle cures, where someone's MS has suddenly vanished and they're claiming it's due to a strange diet, unproven surgery, exercise program or combination of fish oils and vitamin pills. None of these work for everyone, although it's possible some of them have worked for some people. Or maybe their MonSter decided to go into remission for a while. There is a worldwide network of MSers who would pass on information about a cure, if there were one. We're a far more effective conspiracy that anything you might think the drug companies operate to keep good news from us.

An MSer is likely to feel ill most of the time – but we don't always complain about it. There's no point going on and on about a chronic condition that isn't likely to get any better. There's an important difference between being healthy and being happy. If you have a cold, you're miserable for the few days it affects you – but if you lived with it for years, you'd learn to get on with your life regardless. An MSer may be smiling, but it doesn't mean they feel well.

MS is infuriating, frustrating, annoying and depressing. It can cause depression and the symptoms are worsened by negative emotions – but it is NOT caused by them. However weird it may seem, the damage to our central nervous systems can be seen and measured. It's not all in our heads. We're still human beings and we'd like to be treated the same as anyone else. We're hurt when someone refuses to shake hands or call us names in the street. Wouldn't you be?

Many MSers can do things in a small way or for a very short period of time that they can't do for longer. Being able to stand for a minute doesn't mean you can stand for an hour – or even five minutes! Being able to move your legs doesn't mean you can walk unaided. MS doesn't turn us into helpless cripples, but it limits what we can do.

MS affects every part of our lives. Even in remission, we're always taking the MS into account. Will I be okay to attend the wedding next month? How hot is that country when I'd like to visit? Will I have the energy to go out with friends after working all week? Quite simply – we don't know!

Please understand that one of the worst things you can say to someone who's having a bad day is, "But you did it last week!" Many long-term conditions vary from day to day and MS is particularly bad for this. It doesn't mean the MSer is being lazy – it may just mean they need you to be a little more understanding today.

Talking Cure

Worrying is like a rocking horse. It gives you something to do, but it doesn't get you anywhere.

I mention in other chapters that some people assume my medical condition automatically means I want to hear about their problems. And also my concerns that I might inflict my own whinging on other people.

But talking about problems can be healthy, too.

It's really down to how you approach the talking part of a possible cure. The traditional image of a psychiatrist's couch has the "patient" doing most of the talking. As if airing the problems will automatically resolve everything. I don't believe in this. I know plenty of people who will talk all day about their medical complaint / family problems / working difficulties and still have the same problems a week later. And a month later. And ten years later! So what good did talking do?

Please note: I'm not referring to genuine complaints or repeating the same problems to someone who has the power to improve things. I've been in that boat – with a manager who didn't want to hear about the same difficulties he'd heard about last year, even if nothing had been done to improve the situation.

But talking as a cure will only work if you *choose* to make it work. I'm not saying it always works, of course it doesn't – but it will *never* work unless you want it to.

I rarely mention my symptoms to anyone, unless they're relevant in some way or getting worse and giving me a specific problem. Not because I'm embarrassed, but because I don't see the point in burdening anyone else. I do occasionally talk to close friends, if I want to look for a solution to some aspect or other of my worsening MS –

and the friend is practical enough to help without thinking I'm just looking for sympathy.

In fact, the person I talk to most often is my cat. Seriously. She will listen for hours while I explain exactly what the problem is - as long as I keep tickling. And I usually come up with something I can try, or I come to terms with the fact that it ain't gonna get any better. She's a great counsellor, my cat.

Of course, this only works because I've got the kind of brain that is good at problem-solving and if I try to think my way around a problem, there's a good chance an opportunity will appear as I'm describing the obstacle. That's just the way my mind works – and if I can't spot the answer, I have good friends who will try to help.

But when I've tried to help some people in this way, it doesn't always work.

"Sorry I'm late, I overslept," said Mark, dropping his coat onto the chair opposite.

"How've you been? You look exhausted," I asked.

"I am, I guess," he replied. "Saw the specialist at the Royal Gwent yesterday and had to park miles away. You know what the parking's like!"

"Why didn't you get the free bus?"

"I didn't want to wait hours for them to pick me up again," he said.

"And that's worse than walking so far you're like this the next day?"

I know as well as anyone that it's important to maintain your independence, but that doesn't mean refusing help that's available for free when it makes life so much easier. But he still drives himself to all of his appointments and often complains about it. I've given up saying anything, because no-one wants a friend who preaches. But I do think it's worth reserving your limited energy for the important things – and there's no point complaining about the lack of parking at the hospital unless there's a chance of it being improved.

There are various types of talking cures and therapy available. There's a full spectrum of systems, ranging from Cognitive Behavioural Therapy to informal chats with a friend. I've done my share of counselling over the years, not all with disabled people. I've even tried talking about my own problems to someone whose help was offered, but she had an agenda I didn't agree with – and a disregard for my privacy that I find hard to forgive. Unfortunately, there is always a price to be paid. If you can afford it (or get it through the NHS) then it may be helpful to talk about your problems. But if you just want to air the same complaints every week and not work at improving either your situation or your attitude to it, I'd suggest you might not get much benefit.

Underground, Overground

If you're a member of the right age group, you now have a group of furry litter-collectors singing in your head from that title.

"Good Morning, Clearwell Caves. Can I help you?" The man on the phone sounded friendly.

"Hello. I hope you can help. Your website says to ring for details about disabled access," I replied.

"Yes. Were you planning to bring someone in a wheelchair?"

"That's the plan. I'm a wheelchair user and I'd like to visit."

"Well, we always suggest you bring a couple of able-bodied helpers. And the passage gets rather narrow, so big wheelchairs won't fit."

"That's okay, my wheelchair's a lightweight manual one. Does it count if one of the helpers is sitting in the chair?"

"Well, no-one's ever done it with a single helper before. You might like to bring more friends," he suggested.

I've always liked a challenge.

Clearwell Caves are situated in, well under, the Forest of Dean. It's been an active iron mine for 4500 years, and mining equipment is displayed throughout the workings. Although the lowest point in the caves is 100 feet below ground, the access is convenient enough for television crews to use it for filming.

There were four of us in our party: my able-bodied husband Martin and his parents plus me on wheels. Ian, my father-in-law, walks with two sticks and was helped by my mother-in-law, Angela.

The staff were friendly and unfazed by my arriving on wheels. They checked I was not expecting a smooth ride and advised that someone should come back to Reception and ask for assistance if I got stuck!

The underground path is concrete, covered with loose, dusty grit and often narrows to barely wide enough for me to scrape the chair through. There are steep slopes and there isn't much traction for wheels or feet. The occasional metal pipe handrail is provided and I would grab these to pull myself up some slopes or slow myself going down. Where there were no rails, I had to use the raw rock walls. Martin had a tough workout, helping to push me up steep slopes and brake me on the downhill parts.

Clearwell do not claim that their caves are fully accessible, but it is possible to get round in a wheelchair. As they advise, you need two strong people to assist someone in a wheelchair – although one of these can be the wheelchair user themselves. It wouldn't be possible to get around in a chair much wider than 16" in the seat, and I doubt that any powered chairs would fit. But manual wheelchair users with a sense of adventure and an able-bodied friend or two can get around. I have suggested they could offer a certificate to anyone who does complete the circuit in this fashion. There can't be many people who can say they've been 100 feet underground in a wheelchair without the benefit of a lift!

Violet Elizabeth

You're Disabled - Here's my Problem

"What's your problem?" The question came from an elderly woman, leaning over my table in the cafe and pointing at my crutches.

"I have MS," I replied with a shrug. The astute reader will have noticed I get asked this sort of thing quite often and don't make a big deal of it.

"I've got rheumatoid arthritis," she said, making a performance of sitting heavily into the next chair.

"Sorry to hear that," I said, continuing to write the notes I'd been making.

"Yes, it's much worse than what you've got," she continued. And continued. I gave up trying to write as she obviously wasn't going to stop talking about her various aches and pains. She continued while I finished my coffee and was still talking as I pulled myself to my feet and crutches. I still couldn't get a word in edgeways.

"Oh, are you going?" she asked. "I was enjoying our conversation so much..."

I walked away to pay my bill. By the time I left, she'd twisted round in her seat and was aiming her monologue towards the man at the next table. I know she'd gone by the following day, but I can't help wondering if the staff had to push her out the door at closing time.

Now, I know this is really nothing to do with my disability. She just used my crutches as an excuse to strike up a one-sided conversation, but it seems to be a common assumption that anyone with a medical problem is automatically interested in the most mundane (or intimate) details of everyone else's medical complaints. Or maybe they think I've got nothing better to do with my time than sit and listen to their whinges. You know something? I'm not that interested – and I've usually got something better to do.

Don't get me wrong. I've done my share of formal counselling as well as being "Aunty Meggy" to friends, colleagues and relatives. Parts of this book refer to other people's experience of disability as well as my own. But that doesn't mean I'm some sort of listening service. I often wonder if these people ever derive any real benefit from talking so much about their problems. I suspect all they're doing is airing complaints, and don't get any help from what could be cathartic.

Sometimes I wonder if I'm guilty of doing this to people. After all, the definition of a bore is someone who talks incessantly about themselves when you want to talk about yourself. It's very easy to think the other person is dominating the conversation when it's actually a 50:50 split. I decided to put myself to the test.

"Do I talk about my MS much?" I asked.

"All the time," she replied.

"Really? I didn't think I'd said much. What did I mention?"

She thought for a moment. "You were going on and on about how much it hurts today. You're always complaining about the pain. And how difficult it is to do things at home because of your wheelchair."

So now I know it's all about perception. I wasn't in much pain, so I'm sure I hadn't mentioned it. And I don't use my wheelchair at home, so I wouldn't have said that. It's possible I had said something about my MS, but she obviously hadn't been listening. Yet she thought I had been going on about it.

However, I'd heard all the details about her aches and pains. And her neighbours'. And someone I'd never met that she used to work with thirty years ago.

It *is* all about perception. I'm as guilty as anyone of seeing things from my perspective. But I've asked several people if I talk about my MS and what I say about it. It's clear that those who think I talk about it a lot don't actually know anything about the problems it gives me. The close friends I asked all said that I rarely mention it except for relevant practical problems - like asking if they'd checked accessibility at a new restaurant they were recommending. Quite a few said they wanted to ask for more info about my condition but didn't like to ask 'cos I never raised the subject.

So if you think someone's been going on about their problems for the last half hour, ask yourself what they've actually said. If you can remember details, then they probably have been talking about it. If you want to know if you've done the same, ask them if you have, then ask for details.

But please don't assume that anyone with a disability wants to spend an hour listening to your problems, anymore than anyone else.

A Wheelchair is Public Property

"Excuse me – that's my chair," I said, coming out of the plane on my crutches.

"No, it's mine. I'm just waiting for them to take me through customs," replied the grey-haired woman in my wheelchair.

"I'm sorry, but you don't understand. That chair belongs to me," I tried to explain.

"I got here first – you'll have to wait for another one."

The airport staff just stood around, staring at anything except the two of us.

I took a deep breath. "It's not a question of who got here first. That chair is my personal property, it doesn't belong to the airport. If you need assistance, you should have booked it with the airline."

"There's no respect for elders and betters these days," she said, glaring at me. But at least she stood up.

I didn't bother to answer, just sank into the chair, my leg muscles spasming from standing so long in an awkward position.

"You handicapped people are all the same," she called back as she walked away. Quite briskly, too.

This was the worst example, but it's a problem I've encountered several times when flying. Because of my mobility difficulties, I'm always held back on the plane until everyone else has gone. So people think the wheelchair waiting for me is theirs for the taking. If it belongs to the airport, someone just takes it and I have to wait (sat on the floor) until a replacement can be brought. Airport staff won't get involved and they're not allowed to touch a passenger, so if someone sits in my wheelchair, it's up to me to get them out. Luckily, I have a useful travel accessory – my 6'2" husband.

Wheelchairs are very personal items. When you depend on one to get about, you get very attached to them. I paid for a good one, easier for me to push than the usual NHS ones. It also looks a lot better than the boring dull metal standard ones. I give my wheelchair a name and it's a wrench to part with one at replacement time. When you think that I spend more time in my wheels than I do wearing my favourite jeans or carrying my best handbag, you start to see how strong a connection I have with it.

How would you feel if someone picked up your favourite jacket and wore it for ten minutes, 'cos they're cold? Without asking, of course.

When I worked in an office, I would lift myself into my desk chair, leaving the wheelchair next to me. My manager used to borrow it when he wanted to talk to someone, so I had to ask his permission if I needed to go anywhere. I didn't like him doing this, but it's not something you can complain about without sounding petty. I once refused to let a colleague borrow my wheelchair because he'd got to take a server rack to another building and thought it would be easier to push it in my wheelchair than to get someone to help him carry it. He couldn't understand why I didn't want a heavy, oily, angular metal rack in my wheelchair – not to mention being left stranded until he brought it back.

As well as people sitting in the chair, I get annoyed with people who use it in some way, *while I'm sitting there.*

Lots of people think it's acceptable to grab the handles and move a wheelchair, complete with occupant. This can be a stranger barging in front of me in a queue, or a colleague who just thinks it's funny to push me forward a few inches and then jerk me back again. Whatever the reason, moving a wheelchair with me in it is a very dangerous thing to do. I haven't killed anyone yet, but it's only a matter of time.

Then there are the people who assume I'm there to be leant on. Literally. I can't count the number of times I've tried to move off, only to realise someone is leaning on my wheelchair. Sometimes I feel the chair tip as someone rests against the back. I've been sworn at for moving when an elderly man was leaning on my shoulder!

Pregnant ladies complain that strangers will come up to them, touch the bulge and ask "When's it due?" As if the presence of a baby-to-be turns that part of her anatomy into public property.

Well, being in a wheelchair is a bit like being pregnant all over.

Somehow, people feel it's appropriate to pat me on the shoulder, head, knee or anywhere else (sometimes very personal) when they wouldn't dream of doing the same if I was standing up. I've had elderly ladies start combing my hair with their fingers, a man take my glasses off and clean rain off them and even a woman wipe my face with her hanky. I'm perfectly capable of looking after myself – although I'll admit, it's difficult to do any of these when I'm pushing my wheels. Do they assume I'm so helpless? Do they think they're being helpful? Do they feel I'm some sort of dress-up doll? Why don't they ask me if I'd like them to help, instead of just doing it? Whatever their reasoning, they react badly when I ask them to stop.

Another wheelchair-related problem is with people putting things on my chair when I'm out of it. My preference on a train is to scramble out of my wheelchair into a standard seat, which is a much safer way to travel. But this leaves my wheelchair unoccupied and passengers will dump their luggage on top. Most commonly, this is a suitcase dumped on the seat, although one guy wanted to use my chair to hold the front (very muddy) wheel of his mountain bike. Another man tried to lift his case onto the seat, couldn't get it high enough and let it drop onto the footplate instead, lifting the rear wheels off the ground so that the chair was unbraked. In all of these cases, I have to ask the person to remove their luggage, as I may need to use my wheelchair during the trip, (say, to go to the loo). I will not record the kind of responses I get, but they're not what you'd call charitable.

    Now, I've complained elsewhere about the people who won't touch a disabled person, so the reader could rightly point out that I'm being picky here. Shouldn't I be grateful that I'm not being treated as a leper? Well, I don't like being treated differently – whether it's someone refusing to shake hands or someone patting my face as if I'm a dog. And I really don't like people assuming they can use my wheelchair for whatever purpose they feel like. That's a **very** personal bit of property.

No-one Warned Me

There are lots of things that happen as a result of disability.

Firstly, there are the specific physical or mental effects of the condition itself. These are generally easy to find out.

Secondly, there are effects which follow on from the initial symptoms. An obvious one is that a truly sedentary life (and I mean using a wheelchair, not just sitting behind a desk for 40 hours a week) causes constipation. These are harder to find out and no-one warns the patient that they're gonna happen.

Thirdly, there are the social effects. It's well-known that a chronic medical condition puts any relationship under strain and many marriages don't survive the changes. But what about the lesser effects? Here are a few of the details I wish someone had thought to tell me about:

Friendships don't always survive. People aren't sure how to cope when a friend is suddenly struck with an illness or disability. Some people grow closer as a result of this, many more drift apart. It isn't possible to predict which friendships will be strong enough to weather the storm, but people crossing the road to avoid meeting you is a fairly strong sign they don't want you around anymore.

Everyone at work starts to regard you with suspicion. Seriously. Once your diagnosis is known, people start behaving as if you're likely to start foaming at the mouth and biting them. The reactions of colleagues and management tend to be way out of proportion with the impact your condition will actually have at each stage.

In general, people judge you by your disability before anything else. You lose your identity to the illness long before your health fails you.

There is a popular belief that we have passed from the "medical model" of disability to the "social model". I agree with this idea. Basically, it's a statement that we are no longer disabled by the limits of our health as much as we are disabled by the attitude of the society we live in.

Under the medical model, people with chronic health problems were restricted by what they were physically capable of and they understood the logic of their limits.

Under the social model, we are limited by the assumptions and beliefs of other people, which makes it very difficult to understand what those boundaries are – let alone live a full and happy life within them.

But that doesn't mean we have to take it lying down.

You Look So Well!

Warning: Bit of a rant and some rather black humour.

"Meg, hi!"

"Oh, hello. Long time no see."

"How are you? I see you're using the wheelchair now," she continued.

"Ticking over, you know. How are you keeping?"

"Oh, I'm okay. Bit creaky in the joints, back playing up, getting out of breath all the time. So why are you using the wheelchair?"

I shrugged. "Finding it harder to get around, you know."

"But you look so well!"

I can never decide why anyone says this. Is it just a platitude meant to make me feel better? Is it embarrassment at seeing me in my wheelchair? Perhaps it's the British stiff upper lip – never admit someone looks worse than they used to, old boy. Is it an accusation; that I look well and should be running about like everyone else? Perhaps it's just a way to introduce her own various complaints into the conversation.

Or do I actually look well – apart from the fact I'm not walking as well as I used to?

I honestly don't know and I suspect the reasons are different every time I hear those words, but I don't think I ever like hearing them.

I have a premonition that people will walk past my coffin saying, "But she looks so well!"

What is Accessible?

Most people assume that accessibility for disabled people is about being able to get a wheelchair into the venue, having a toilet big enough to accommodate a wheelchair and ramps where necessary for a person in a wheelchair. Yet not all disabled people are wheelchair users.

Accessibility can mean Braille letters on lift buttons; a hearing loop system to aid those with hearing aids; a sign language interpreter at a theatre and innumerable other adaptations to make services available to those who have a disability.

Let's be honest, it isn't possible to cater for everyone! So businesses have to compromise between desirability and reality.

Speaking for myself, I generally ask if a venue is wheelchair accessible. It's easier than explaining what I can and can't do if I'm on crutches - and I'm increasingly likely to be on wheels, anyhow. If I am on crutches, I can manage a few steps– it's actually easier for me to get up one high step than two smaller ones, unless they're far apart. I can cope with a non-disabled loo, subject to a few adaptations – in other words, I can't manage in a "normal" one. I'll spare you the details.

I find some venues place restrictions on me more than those imposed by my condition. One restaurant refused to admit me, because they didn't think I could get out quickly enough in the case of a fire. I've also known a theatre tell me I can't keep my crutches with me, as they'd be an obstruction to other people if there were a fire. (And me being unable to walk is *less* of an obstruction?)

Ideally, service providers should discuss the needs and restrictions of a disabled person with that person, coming to an agreement regarding what is possible, what is safe and what cannot be done. But in the real world, they make assumptions and we have to live with them.

Each of us has a different set of requirements, so the onus is on the disabled person to ask the right questions and make their needs clear. We're all embarrassed about it, but it's better to discuss it over the phone beforehand than turn up on the day and find out you've had a wasted journey. I have a standard list of questions to ask when I need to check out a new venue – and clear ways of explaining what I need. It's actually getting easier as I rely more on my wheelchair – people tend to assume a person on crutches can stand indefinitely and walk as far as anyone else.

If there's somewhere locally you'd like to go that isn't accessible, or if your condition is worsening and you're afraid you won't be able to manage the step, talk to the management and see what can be done. Our local Italian restaurant has a single, high step at the door. I can park my buggy immediately outside and then manage on my crutches and it's fine once I'm inside – there's even an accessible loo on the ground floor. But I'm aware that it's getting harder for me to walk on crutches and the day will come when I'll be on wheels. I spoke to the manager, feeling very embarrassed. It's always awkward to admit to someone that my symptoms are getting worse and to broach the subject of access.

"It's not a problem," he assured me.

"But – the step," I replied.

"I can get you up the step. We've had wheelchairs in here before."

And that was it. No fuss, no arguing – just a simple statement that Carmine would get me in.

It's nice to feel wanted.

I know I've mentioned this elsewhere in the book, but a willing hand is worth more than three ramps. And if it comes with a genuine smile, it's worth a dozen!

What is a Symptom?

A straightforward question that gets more complicated as you look into it.

Any dictionary will provide a definition of the word symptom along the lines of a "perceptible change from normal function, sensation or appearance" due to a chronic illness, for example. Although the definition is correct, it demonstrates that "symptom" is a hard concept to pin down. Define "perceptible" and "normal" for a start! Add the unpredictable nature of MS to the equation and the confusion increases dramatically. There are three main areas of confusion around symptoms.

Firstly: what constitutes a perceptible change? The symptoms of MS are so variable and unpredictable that it's hard to be certain about changes. Is my walking worse than it was six months ago? Am I *unreasonably* tired at the end of a working day? Has this odd feeling in my arm only occurred since I've had MS? Every MSer experiences moments of doubt, wondering whether something is a genuine symptom – or a coincidence.

Secondly: what is caused by MS? And how directly – is it specifically a symptom of MS or of something else caused by the MS? Or is it nothing to do with the MS, just coincidental?

Thirdly: will the medical profession accept it as a symptom?

The first problem is best tackled by use of an MS diary. It's worthwhile noting down new symptoms when they occur, together with brief details about its circumstances, severity and duration. This doesn't have to be onerous, something along the lines of:
Felt suddenly tired this afternoon, could hardly lift my

head off the desk. Came on about an hour after air-conditioning failed at work.

It's amazing how easy it is to spot patterns (like heat causing fatigue) can be spotted in such a diary. Not to mention its usefulness in recording new problems. A notebook or computer file is all that's needed – just make a note of changes. Don't forget to record something returning to normal (that word again!).

Addressing the issue of whether something is caused directly by MS, as a result of something caused by the MS or is completely unrelated can be complicated. The common symptoms of MS are well-documented and it's probably reasonable to assume that an MSer who experiences something off this list can safely blame it on the MonSter. Unless they suffer from something with similar symptoms– in which case, does it matter what causes the problem? However, it can be beneficial to certain symptoms with a non-MS specialist. My GP arranged a series of blood tests when I asked about my fatigue, which identified the fact that I have pernicious anaemia. A course of iron tablets and regular B12 injections keep it under control, so any remaining fatigue is due to the MonSter.

The medical profession, including many MS specialists and other neurological staff, rely heavily on the list I mentioned above. They seem to be reluctant to call something a symptom unless it has been identified as such for many years. For example, a conversation between myself and a Neurologist.

Me: "I've noticed my food allergies have got worse, can that be down to the MS?"

Neuro: "No, that isn't caused by the MS."

Me: "Okay, just thought I'd ask."

Neuro: "I've heard several MS patients say the same thing, but it's just a coincidence."

Now, I accept that it isn't on "the list", but isn't it relevant that it's been reported by other patients? Maybe a common problem like this would be worth investigating - if the medical profession would record its occurrences. If we only record the symptoms we already know about, we may be missing that vital piece of information that will lead to an explanation of the condition. Maybe even a cure!

Trust Me, I'm a Doctor

No, not me! I'm strictly an amateur with a vested interest!

But I've learnt to be cynical about all members of that strange tribe we call doctors. Yes, they can do a lot of good and I certainly couldn't cope without their help. But they aren't omniscient and they sometimes make mistakes. Cases of doctors abusing their patients' trust are, thankfully, rare – although the press likes to make the most of such incidents. But, there is something I always bear in mind whenever I deal with a doctor:

They all used to be medical students.

It's much harder to be overawed by someone if you think about them as one of those beer-swilling, prank-playing teenagers.

On a more serious note, it's important to remember that doctors are only human and as fallible as the rest of us. They do make mistakes and the wise patient will keep that in mind at all times.

Having said all that, I am fortunate to have the support of some great doctors. This is not just luck, there are ways to find a good doctor and then maximise the benefits of your relationship. And it is a relationship, believe me.

The best way to locate a new doctor is to shop around. When I move into a new area, I register with a GP practice that has several doctors listed. Then, each time I need to see one, I choose a different name from the list. Until I find one that "clicks". So far, I've always managed to find a GP I like. They're not as rare as some people think – you just have to look for them.

So how do I decide if that doctor's right for me? Well, I turn up with a short list of things I want to mention

– all for the same problem, as the appointment isn't an hour long. If s/he seems interested, willing to talk and not put off by my list, we're over the first hurdle. Then it helps if we get on with each other. Most people with chronic conditions know more about their own condition than any General Practitioner will know and it's important they recognise this fact. I'm not saying I know more than a doctor about everything, only about some aspects of *my* problems.

A little scenario:

"So how can I help you, today?" asked my doctor.

"Well, I've been suffering with more muscle spasms, and wondered if we could do anything about it," I replied.

"Difficult. There are plenty of drugs on the market, but they're very strong and the side-effects can be bad."

"I know; I've been doing some research. There's this new one, which might work without turning me into a zombie," I hand over my notebook, with the name of the new drug printed carefully in block letters.

"I haven't heard of this one. Let's look it up..."

Now, I would never try to bully a doctor into prescribing something they think is wrong for me – but I'm very happy to go into the consulting room with info I've gleaned from other sources. The internet can be a good source, especially some of the online communities. Some charities publish news about new treatments on the market, occasionally they're even reported in the mainstream media. Wherever I hear about them, I do my research and then discuss it with a doctor. I've never disagreed with my doctor about treatments, but I've never asked for anything expensive or experimental, either. We work as a team and my health is much better because of this.

As an MSer, the Neurology department of my local hospital is a major factor in my care. I have regular appointments with my Neurologist and can make an appointment to see the MS Specialist Nurse at reasonably short notice. When I moved house, I stayed with the same team, as they're just as close as the hospital I would now be assigned to – and they're a top-notch research facility. Patient choice works! (Well, this time, anyhow.) This is another relationship that benefits both of us. I get excellent NHS care and the team get a willing participant in their research projects.

There have been occasions when I have needed to see specialists in other fields, due to some of the MonSter's other symptoms. In each case, I begin by approaching my GP or Neurologist about the problem and asking them to refer me as they think fit. I approach my first meeting with a new specialist in the same way – work out what I need to tell them about and make a short list of details to mention. A short-term problem may mean I only need to see them once or twice, but it's worth working on the relationship from the start. And treating them like a human being, not just a machine for writing prescriptions.

Boys Don't Make Passes

... at girls who wear glasses, as the saying goes. They're even less likely to find someone attractive if they're in a wheelchair.

Seriously, dating is difficult for a disabled person. One young man I know in an online community asked the question, "If I'm going out with a girl – when do I mention my MS?" Since his disability isn't obvious, he's going to have to tell her at some point. But when? I think it's a question that can only be answered on an individual basis – when you feel you know each other quite well, but early enough so she doesn't feel you were keeping her in the dark. Personally, I thought he was wrong to say he was going to start each conversation at a speed-dating event by telling the girl that he had MS, but it's his decision.

I've often come across people who will flirt with everyone *except* the one in the wheelchair. Judging by reactions, most people assume that anyone with a disability doesn't have a sex life and must be treated differently. Believe me, being in a wheelchair does not automatically turn us into prudes.

It is true, a wheelchair is one of the most unflattering fashion accessories ever designed. I sometimes refer to my purple-framed, lightweight wheelchair as "sexy" – but that's in relation to the clunky, heavy ones issued by the NHS. Having fabric bunched up your lap and a skirt wrapped tightly to keep it away from the wheels is not a good look.

There are suppliers of clothing especially for wheelchair users, but these are expensive and look, shall we say, utilitarian - even boring. High Street fashion is certainly not designed for people who spend their lives sitting down. It's even harder for those of us who use the wheelchair some of the time but can stand up as well. We haven't got a hope!

My own solution is to buy "normal" clothing, which looks okay when I'm on my crutches and I keep the extra bulk in my lap as neat as I can when I'm the wheelchair. A handbag helps to hide it, too. When I try clothes on, I check their appearance when I'm sitting down as well as standing up (something most changing rooms aren't equipped for). I avoid bracelets and flowing sleeves as these tend to snag and / or break. It means there are some things I just can't wear, but it's not too bad. I tend to wear colours, rather than neutral tones – partly because I like to, but also to make a statement. I'd rather not blend into the background and the wheelchair makes me hard enough to see, anyway. It's also easier for people who don't like to say the "double-u word". I've heard this sort of comment several times, when someone needs to point me out:

"She's that one – the woman in the w-..."

They can't finish that word. I mean, isn't it discrimination? What if I'm offended to hear them mention that I'm in a wheelchair? So I dress in a way that gives them an acceptable alternative:

"She's over there – the one in the purple hat."

Or hippy waistcoat, or colourful knitted jacket, or whatever.

Just because I'm disabled doesn't mean I have to be boring.

Admittedly, I could be wearing a set of flashing lights and some people would still ignore me – see *Cloak of Invisibility*. But no-one can say I don't try to be visible.

As well as clothing, simple things like putting on make-up or shaving can be a major problem for those with limited hand function or sensitivity. It's another area where we each have to make our own decision. I rarely wear makeup, as it's difficult for me to apply, but others wouldn't leave the house without their face on. I know at least one MSer who reckons the only reason he sports a full beard is because he's scared his hand will slip when he's shaving!

I have met men who find the idea of a woman in a wheelchair attractive *because* of the wheelchair. I don't know if it's the idea that she's somehow helpless that appeals, but it seems a little odd to me. Whether it's a turn-off or a turn-on, surely the wheelchair shouldn't be what's important?

There have been campaigns with slogans like, "See the person – not the wheelchair", one of which featured a photo of a very attractive young lady in a wheelchair – stark naked. I I'm not about to try this and I'm sure there are people who still wouldn't notice me if I did.

Blaming the Victim

Many years ago, I learnt how to break up a fight or prevent an argument coming to blows:

You move the least aggressive person out of the fight.

Now, while this works well for fights in bars, it's not always applicable in other scenarios – such as bullying situations, where it may not be reasonable to do this.

For example, I was on a week-long training course, where one person on the course exhibited increasingly nasty behaviour towards me. Worried about what might happen, I had reported this repeatedly to the staff in charge, who'd dismissed my concerns. They told me others had commented on the behaviour of this particular man, so it was nothing to do with my disability. As if that somehow made it alright! Until an overt, anonymous, threat was made towards me, when they insisted I call my husband to take me home. I didn't want to leave, but they promised me a full refund and a replacement course as soon as it could be arranged.

Remove the least aggressive person and everyone's happy.

Except the one who's been on the receiving end of the threats and has to leave. It cost me the remainder of the course, a day's leave for Hubby and a lot of hurt.

Now, I accept that the aggressor could easily be a disabled person, so it isn't exactly discrimination to send the bullied person home. But it's more likely that the target will be the one in the wheelchair. Or with the hearing aids. Or whatever it is that sets them apart. I suspect the staff would have promised me anything to get me to leave. Maybe this is their preferred way of dealing with bullying on a course. Whatever the reasons, I felt I'd been treated badly.

This is a particularly bad example, but it's not the only time I've been punished for being the victim. By choosing to take part in activities alongside non-disabled people, it could easily be said that I'm setting myself up as a target for bullies and other people who think it's appropriate to single out anyone who's different. If I'd chosen to attend a course specifically tailored for disabled people, then the situation might have been different. Organisers often suggest this alternative, to reduce the risk of "personality clashes" they may have to deal with. But don't I have the right to choose the course I feel is appropriate to my skills and aspirations? Rather than the one for which the only qualification is a disability?

When bullying is done anonymously, it's even more usual for the target to be "punished" as it's easier than identifying the perpetrators. So those who think disabled people belong in a sort of ghetto and that wheelchair users should live in "special" hospitals get their wish, by forcing us out of mainstream society.

There's a lot more to making work places, courses and service accessible than just installing a ramp. Sometimes it's necessary for those in charge to stand up for someone's rights, too.

The Rules of Complaining

Despite all my moans in this book, I'm generally pretty easy-going and don't complain very often. Although I could have done, I've never sued anyone for discrimination, although that may change. We never know what the future holds.

If I complained about every little act of discrimination, I'd never get anything else done. Whether it's the customer service person who speaks LOUDLY and s-l-o-w-l-y when I admit to having a disability or the shop assistant who serves the woman behind me instead of me, it's just not worth it. But every now and then, I've had enough and a complaint is lodged. Generally, it's because something truly outrageous has happened and I want a resolution or at least some assurance that it won't happen to someone else. Occasionally it's a relatively small incident, but I've just HAD ENOUGH!

Ahem.

Storming out of a shop, yelling that you'll see them in court may make you feel better, but it's not doing any good if you don't intend to follow through. You'll only reinforce their view that disabled people are troublemakers.

So. I've decided I'm going to make a complaint. Once thing I know for sure is that there's no point just shouting and screaming about it. I need to find the appropriate recipient for my complaint and make sure I present myself in the right manner.

Rule 1: Find the appropriate target.
Sometimes a complaint should be directed to the person who you think is at fault. A simple, "I'm sorry, what did you call me?" may be enough to make them reconsider their position. More usually, a complaint needs to be aimed higher. Ask to see the shop's duty manager or write to the

company's Head Office. It may be better to send the complaint to an outside body. Is there an Ombudsman covering this type of business? Would a letter to the local paper get the Council's attention?

Rule 2: Be honest.

Tempting though it is to exaggerate, the truth is your best weapon. The sales assistant knows she didn't use any four-letter words, so don't claim she did – stick to the truth and say it's inappropriate for her to push your wheelchair to move you out of her way.

Rule 3: Put it in writing.

Only the most minor of complaints will be dealt with verbally. A written complaint stands a better chance of being dealt with appropriately than a verbal one. It doesn't necessarily have to be a letter – an email may suffice. If it doesn't, send a letter – recorded delivery if you have to.

Rule 4: Don't lose your temper.

Trust me, it won't do any good at all. I've mentioned occasions when I've thrown my toys out of the pram or shouted at people to get their attention. But these actions are only to be avoided if possible. I'm not acting or "putting it on" when I shout at people!

Rule 5: Know what you want.

Don't complain just for the sake of it. If you can't think of something you want to get from this situation, then you're wasting your time. It may be compensation or it may be a simple apology, but you need to know exactly what you hope to achieve.

Rule 6: Be prepared to negotiate.

You may ask for compensation for your damaged wheelchair, they may offer to pay the repair bill instead. You may want to see the sales assistant prostrate himself in apology for his rudeness, but you'll have to settle for a mumbled "Sorr-ee" instead. Think of it as taking the moral high ground and being magnanimous when you compromise in this way.

Rule 7: Give them every chance to respond.
Allow time for your letter to be read and replied to. Remember the manager dealing with it will need to speak to the employee you're complaining about. If you don't get a reply to your first letter, send another one by recorded delivery and add a note that you're expecting them to compensate you for having to do so.

Rule 8:Keep records.
Keep copies of receipts, letters you send, details of phone calls made, people spoken to, etc. After a recent experience with an organisation who've refused to meet their obligations after months of phone calls and letters, I'm starting to think I need to keep records of every "official" phone call I ever make. It's a sorry world.

Rule 9: Know your rights.
If you don't know your rights, keep quiet until you can find out. The internet is a good place to look them up. Or your local library. If it turns out they don't have to accommodate you – take your custom where it's appreciated.

Rule 10: Keep the law out of it unless you have no choice.
Seriously, taking someone to court is a serious matter and you need to be sure you really want to put that much time and energy into your complaint. If you're not, swallow your pride and move on.

This may look like a long list, but it's really just common sense.

Keep calm.
Be more reasonable than they are.
Know what you want to achieve.
And – good luck.

The Only Certainty

Warning: This chapter includes straight talk about death and subjects that we, as Brits, don't like to talk about. I'm going to discuss wills and donor cards (and explain why I have two of each) as well as funerals and the importance of discussing these taboo subjects with your nearest and dearest.

"*Certainty? In this world nothing is certain but death and taxes.*" Benjamin Franklin.

Sorry to argue, Mr Franklin. But it's possible to live without paying taxes. It's even legal in the State of Alaska!

No-one can cheat death, though.

It isn't a comfortable thought, but eventually each of us will die. In some Western cultures, we've become very squeamish about it. Death happens in hospitals and care homes; rarely at home, surrounded by family. We never see a dead body and we think they're somehow disgusting; so we pay strangers to look after our loved ones' remains. I'm not suggesting we revive the curious 19th Century custom of photographing our dead relatives seated in the parlour. But this reluctance to discuss death causes all sorts of problems.

Every year, thousands of UK citizens die without leaving a will. Family members bicker over their inheritance and most of them end up feeling cheated. The only person who can be sure of getting a fair share is the taxman. (Maybe Ben Franklin was right, after all.) How can anyone be sure who Grandad wanted to inherit his books and fishing tackle? Did Aunty Edna want her family to have her savings or would she rather have it go to the hospice that eased her last months? The laws governing inheritance aren't as simple as people expect – and sometimes everything goes to the Government by default. A basic will needn't cost much and a free service is sometimes available from local solicitors; or charities who hope to benefit. If we can get over our squeamishness enough to write our wishes down.

A friend once explained how he'd been diagnosed with a terminal condition and told he had between six months and a year to live. Once he'd got over the shock, he made a list of things to do with his remaining months. He went through his writing and photographs, organising, throwing out drafts and writing an index. He visited friends and relatives he hadn't seen for years. He patched up old feuds and did many of the things we'd all like to do in that situation. Then he realised his condition wasn't getting any worse. He went back to the specialists and they repeated the tests, eventually admitting they'd made a mistake with his diagnosis. I heard this story more than five years afterwards, when he explained that he'd actually felt a little disappointed to be told he was going to live. After resigning himself to his fate and deciding to make the most of his last months, he found it hard to re-adjust to a normal, uncertain future. But when the Grim Reaper eventually comes calling, that's one man who'll be ready to face him.

Obviously, it's never easy to hear you only have a few months to live. But there is that silver lining. Most of us never think about our own mortality until we're confronted with it – which is one reason a terminal diagnosis comes as such a shock. A little forward planning can ease the blow for everyone.

As mentioned above, I have a formal will. It's not complicated, but it will make sure what I leave behind goes where I want it to. And not where I don't.

I also have a *Living Will*. A document that details the care I want to receive if I'm unable to make or express my own decisions, for any reason. These documents, also known as *Advance Care Directives,* are becoming more common, as medical science improves and people begin to wonder about the quality of their life, as well as how many years they may have left. A quick search of the internet produces a few websites which offer free downloadable templates for living wills. (Search for *Living Will Free Template*, which will also list a lot of sites offering to write them for money.) If you do go for the DIY approach - keep it simple, get it witnessed and discuss it with your family and friends. The easiest option is to nominate someone to make decisions if you're unable to do so, rather than trying to second-guess every possible situation that might occur. By all means, record your choices about treatments, but the important thing is to give someone you trust a *Power of Attorney*, should you become incapacitated. Many factors influence the contents of a living will, including your personal beliefs (religious or otherwise) and the likely progression of any chronic condition. Decisions are easier to make before they become critical; and worth recording for the time when they're needed.

As I mentioned above, I carry two donor cards. I used to give blood on a regular basis and received my silver award for 25 donations before I was diagnosed with MS. Although I'm no longer allowed to give blood, I'm still registered on the UK Transplant donor database; so that my kidneys, heart, etc. can be used for transplant or research. More information is available at: www.uktransplant.org.uk or ask your GP.

The second donor card is for the UK Multiple Sclerosis Tissue Bank. My registration with them states that they are welcome to use the parts of my body affected by MS (basically my central nervous system and a few other tissues) for research purposes after I'm dead. If research into neurological conditions like MS is to progress, it's vital that scientists have these for research and I'm happy to think I can help in one last way. For anyone who's interested, their website is: www.ukmstissuebank.imperial.ac.uk and they need **non-MSers** as well as MSers on the register.

Organ donation is a difficult subject and many people have concerns about registering. If this is the case, the websites listed above will help, offering useful information and contact details for people you can speak to. For anyone who doesn't like the idea of their organs being used in this way, I would ask a simple question: *Would you accept a donated organ if you or someone you love needed it?* If your answer is "Yes" – then shouldn't you be on the donor register? Organ donation in the UK is currently based on an "opt-in" register, so you need to specifically ask to be added as a potential donor. However, at the time of writing, the Welsh Assembly Government has finished a public consultation on organ donation. They say that the majority of responders prefer an "opt-out" system, so that anyone who *doesn't* want to participate has to register that fact. I heartily support this proposed change and hope that Wales' lead is followed by the rest of the UK and other countries.

And finally, funerals. It may be hard to think about, but every decision you make about your own funeral is one less for your loved ones to think about – at a time when they've got enough to deal with. You can't exactly insist that everyone should enjoy your funeral, but there are requests you can make in advance. Do you have a preference for a church service or a civil one? Music you'd like to be played? Photographs to be displayed? Friends who should be invited? Perhaps a charity you'd like to nominate in case people wish to make donations?

There's no reason you can't ask for something different. Some people record their own eulogy or a message for those who'll be gathered for the funeral. A slide show of happier times, perhaps. I've yet to see a PowerPoint presentation – but I'm sure it's been done. Do you have a friend you'd like to speak about you? Maybe not the way John Cleese spoke at Graham Chapman's memorial service, though. Unless that's what you'd like.

There's also the difficult question of paying for a funeral. Like weddings, there is no upper limit to the amount you can pay and even a basic service will cost several hundred pounds. A few company pension schemes pay a contribution towards funeral costs. Some people arrange a Funeral Plan - a sort of savings scheme that covers the cost of a basic funeral and cremation. Others make provision in their wills, assuming they'll leave enough money to cover it and this is a good place to mention whatever arrangement you have, rather than leaving money worries for your loved ones. In cases of genuine hardship, there is the possibility of a one-off payment from the Social Fund in the UK, details are available through your Job Centre or the Local Council.

I've been to all kinds of funerals – it's inevitable with my large extended family and circle of friends. I've seen an organist almost fall off his seat when he realised how loudly our massed family will sing *Cwm Rhondda*; I've watched a wicker coffin carried into a memorial woodland for anonymous burial; I've heard all sorts of hymns, popular songs, poems and even birdsong played during the ceremony. Sometimes flowers are welcome, sometimes donations to a charity are preferred. At one funeral, no-one was allowed to wear black. Writing this chapter has brought back many happy memories, as well as a few tears. We can all hope to be remembered that way.

The Rainbow and other happy places

Happy Places

"It's a private network," said a voice over my shoulder.

"Sorry?" I asked, twisting in my seat to see who was speaking,

"You can't logon to our network. It's private."

"Erm, I'm not trying to. I was just doing some writing," I replied.

"You can't do it on our network!" She was getting annoyed with me now.

I sighed. "Look, I'm not trying to connect to a network. I'm writing something on my laptop. That's all."

"What are you writing?" She leaned in front of me, looking at my screen.

"Excuse me!" Now I was annoyed and I closed my laptop. She walked away and I saw her talking to another member of staff, pointing in my direction. He came over.

"I'm sorry, you can't use that in here," he said.

"Pardon?"

"We don't give access to customers, it's for staff use only."

"Look, as I explained to your colleague, I'm not trying to use your network. I'm just writing something on my laptop. Working offline," I tried to keep my tone level and probably failed.

"It doesn't matter what you say you're doing, you can't use that in here."

Now, I assume that buying a coffee give me the right to sit and type quietly in a café for half an hour. I wasn't using their network, I hadn't plugged in to a mains socket – I couldn't understand their problem at all. I think I do now. On another occasion, I was reading a book in the same café. A member of staff kicked my crutches over (which were propped against the table) and cleared away my half-drunk coffee. She then stood and stared at me until I left. Speaking to other disabled people in the town, I find they've had similar experiences. The café advertises how pensioner-friendly it is and actively encourages teenagers, but apparently doesn't see the need to be nice to disabled customers. Maybe we're not good for the image it wants to project.

Fortunately, there is another café in town which is far more friendly. By a strange coincidence,it's are called The Rainbow (nothing to do with this book, honest!). Maybe I should have arranged a sponsorship deal...

Anyway, The Rainbow don't care if a customer is disabled. They're happy for me to buy a coffee and type for an hour – with free use of their WiFi network, if I want it.

Since retiring from full-time employment, I've experienced all sorts of reactions to my disability. From the abrupt behaviour of staff at one café to the welcome I receive at another one, with all shades in between. I can't be sure how much of this is due to my disability, of course – it's possible people are confused by an adult who's neither looking after children nor rushing off to work. But I think it's the disability, to be honest.

Of course, there are groups I've only met because of my disability. Groups like Disability Arts Cymru, the Women's Arts Association and various offshoots of MS charities. There are other groups that I've come into contact with as a writer – and my writing has only happened because I had to retire from full-time work. Adult education bodies, especially those that provide weekend courses, such as Farncombe Estate in the Cotswolds. As I come to the end of writing this book, I realise I've talked far more about the bad things that happen to disabled people than the positive aspects. That's partly because the negative events are the ones that stick in the mind but mostly because they're the important ones for me to document.

To set the record straight, I must stress that many places genuinely welcome disabled people and most people are perfectly friendly to someone in a wheelchair. I've named a few in the course of this book, but there are many I haven't mentioned and far more that I haven't met. I hope that the day will come when venues that fail to meet the needs of disabled customers will be as rare as "Whites Only" signs. Until then, I will continue to seek out my own happy places.

The Printed Word

I have this image in my head, of myself in the not-so-distant future. I'm sitting in a circle of mismatched plastic chairs in a dingy room. Most of the other chairs are occupied, with an odd mixture of people. There's a man who looks like a retired academic and a couple of homeless people surrounded with bulging plastic bags. A young, unshaven man sits restlessly as his hand reaches toward a suspicious-looking bulge in his coat pocket. A lady in a business suit sits very upright in her chair, avoiding eye contact with everyone else. And there's me. I raise my hand for silence; then say,

"My name is Meg and I'm a bookaholic."

It's true – I've been addicted to the printed word since I first learnt to read. I devour books; I review them for a couple of magazines; I have boxes of them piled up at home. (My Hubby says we moved house to make room for the books. I *think* he's joking!) I just can't resist books, and now I'm writing them, too. There's no hope – I will have to found Bookaholics Anonymous.

In light of this confession, it will come as no surprise that I love libraries. I can still remember the joy I felt when I learnt our local village library held only the smallest fraction of the books in the world. I'd read everything in the children's section, and the Librarian suggested she could order me some more from other libraries. Until then I'd assumed their shelves held everything in existence!

I'm still the same. The staff in our town library greet me by name, as do the local bookshops. The world of books seems to be full of people who have no problem with my disability. Whether I'm reaching for a high shelf, struggling to carry books because of my crutches, or stacking a pile of them on my lap in my wheelchair, there's always someone who's willing to lend a hand. I don't know what it is about people who read, but I feel welcomed in a bookshop or library.

In recent years, I've gained a third reason for being in libraries. As well as reading the books and writing them, I present creative writing workshops, and local libraries are keen to use me for this. I take a particular delight from these workshops, because of the mix of people they attract. There are usually a few people from a local writing group, one or two pensioners writing their memoirs, a schoolchild keen to learn and the odd frustrated poet. There may even be a few disabled people, too. Writing is a true equal-opportunities environment, and one that many people with chronic illnesses have discovered. Very few of them know that I'm disabled myself, until they first meet me – which is how I like it. Although I write about disability issues and sometimes present workshops specifically for groups of writers with disabilities, I don't consider my disability to be relevant to most of my writing. I write as a human being, with all of my experience of the world, and my health issues are no more important than the colour of my skin or my gender.

But it isn't just the book world. I've heard similar stories from other disabled people, about people who share their own interests and I've come to the conclusion that most people are more comfortable with a disabled person if there is a reason for their being together. It's human nature to judge fellow enthusiasts (in whatever field) more generously than we do people we meet at random. It's a reassuring observation for people who become disabled, that the people who share their passions are likely to welcome them as they always have. Even the direct impact of a disability is lessened by this behaviour, when others are willing to make accommodation. There are hugely active communities of disabled motorcyclists, sportspeople, ramblers, musicians and many other interests - a disability does not have to mean the end of someone's lifelong passion for their hobby. In many cases they can continue to participate with the same able-bodied people they've known for years.

The best piece of advice I can offer someone who's worried that their disability means an end to their participation in whatever activity they love is to *try*. Many (but admittedly not all) problems can be overcome if the participant and their associates are willing to try. If no-one tries, nothing is ever achieved. And continuing in our chosen activities is an important part of our humanity. Sorry to preach, but it's a truth that isn't as obvious to some people as I'd like it to be.

So – anyone want to join Bookaholics Anonymous?

The Virtual World

The internet has brought so much to many people's lives, especially disabled people. I don't have to leave the house or even pick up a phone to chat to a friend when I want company. I can access reference material and detailed information about anything I want to, without stirring from my comfy seat. The online world may be a scary place at first, much like moving to a new city where the roadsigns are in a foreign language and the inhabitants are all rushing past on their way somewhere. But the language is easy to learn and there are always friendly people willing to help a newbie (newcomer!).

There are also hazards in so-called cyber-space, just as in the real world. Anyone venturing onto the internet should look into all-round security software from a reputable supplier – just as you would lock your car before leaving it outside a shop. Never give out personal information if you don't want it widely known. Never, *ever,* give your bank details unless you know who's going to see them. A little caution is always better than a lot of regrets. Most people have a family member or neighbour who'll help them get started on the web. Or try contacting your local library. Much though I mourn the passing of quiet libraries full of books, they've become a good place for many people to make their first small journeys on the information superhighway.

So what's the point of the internet, especially for someone with a chronic health problem? Simply, it's a way to communicate. It doesn't replace real-world interactions, just adds a few new ones. So you can keep in touch with someone by popping round for a cuppa, phoning them for a chat, sending them a letter – and now by email, chat rooms, social networking and a host of other online methods. Just as in the real world, you start by finding sites for people with similar interests – in my case reading, writing, knitting and so on. It's very easy to build a social circle in this way and there are many people I count as friends that I've never met – and probably never will.

There are also sites aimed specifically at disabled people. Some of these have a forum or message boards where users can exchange messages with each other. In theory, these are welcoming, supportive groups where everyone is in the same boat and individuals can be open about their problems and discuss possible solutions in a friendly environment. Sometimes it works – but not always. One site may have a political agenda, another may be encouraging benefit fraud by discussing how to cheat the system. Some sites are dominated by a clique of users, who push their views at newcomers and gang up on dissenting voices. I've known a few that are just whinge-fests where people post their complaints and everybody agrees with them. If you join a site and find it just doesn't suit you, then don't go back. You haven't paid for anything, you don't owe them anything and you don't have much chance of changing the established culture of a site. Just go looking for another one – or ask an online buddy if they know of one. You wouldn't keep going to a pub that's full of football fans every Saturday when you want to watch the rugby, so don't waste your time on a website that doesn't suit your likes, either.

The anonymity of the internet allows people to behave in a way they would never do face-to-face. This is great if you want to ask if anyone else has the same embarrassing symptom as you, but it also means some individuals will take advantage of their untraceability. If it happens to you or you see unacceptable comments aimed at another user, report it to the site's Admins

(Administrators). Just as in the real world, cyber-bullying is everyone's problem.

There are other forms of bullying, too. People who have disabilities can be as racist, sexist or outright rude as anyone else, but may feel that their disability gives them a licence to express these views. As before, if you don't like people's behaviours, try another site.

Sites aimed at disabled people have a particular problem that I've never seen anywhere else. A new user appears in the forum and posts something like:

> Hello everyone. I'm a student at Erehwon University and I need your help with this term's project. I have to find out about disabled people, so I'd like you all to tell me about your experiences of being disabled.

Sometimes these posters ask more specific questions or phrase their request more politely; sometimes they are a lot less grammatical than my example. If you wish to do their work for them, be my guest. If you wish to "flame" them for assuming you've got nothing better to do with your time, you're also welcome to do so. If you prefer to track them down and throw a brick through their window, please don't!

Occasionally there are respectable surveys carried out online, but it's obvious when it's just someone looking for easy answers to their homework designed to improve their awareness of minority groups. I applaud the idea that education should encourage students to connect with disabled people – but this is not the way to go about it. Many sites have stated policies that such behaviour is not tolerated, in which case you could just report it to the Admins. As with everything else, if you're not happy – move on. There are lots more sites out there and there will be others that you're more comfortable with.

(As an aside, I've been asked on several occasions if I will agree to being interviewed for such research and have been happy to help, both online and in the meat-world. This isn't an invitation for everyone to contact me, just a suggestion that many of us would help, if approached properly.)

Many non-disability sites have more disabled people using them than you'd find in a random group, simply because the internet is accessible. You'll also find lots of unemployed people, stay-at-home parents and anyone else who may have more time to spend on a computer.

One word of warning – I was an active member of a writing website where users would post their work for critique and comment on others' stories. Actually, I've been on quite a few of these, but this is about one particular site. There was an active social forum on there and I joined in with this side of things, as well as becoming a much-requested critic. I never mentioned my disability as I didn't think it was relevant. Then I posted a story told from the point of view of a wheelchair user and got some nasty comments from other site members who objected to me claiming to know how a disabled person thought. I took a deep breath and decided to admit that I am disabled, but was flamed by those who'd decided I was pretending. One of the site Admins suggested I should post an apology if I couldn't "prove" I was disabled, so I left the site. There are as many small-minded people on the internet as anywhere else and always a few looking for something to take offence at.

So welcome to the internet – some weeks I feel like I spend more time on here than I do in the real world. Usually it's a fun place to be and I look forward to bumping into you there.

Prescribed Exercise and Other Programs

A couple of years ago, there was a local scheme where GPs could refer patients for regular exercise sessions. I heard about it and asked to be "prescribed" onto it.

I had to go to our local leisure centre twice a week to take part in a mild form of circuit training. We didn't use any gym machines, but portable equipment like gym balls, steps and hand weights. A circuit of gentle exercises was set up and participants worked round the room, spending two minutes at each station. It's surprisingly good exercise and the mixed group of attendees mostly seemed to get something out of it.

But there were problems with the scheme. Few of us had done any formal exercise since we were at school and we didn't know how to do things like hamstring stretches or triceps curls. There wasn't as much explanation as some people needed and even less help for those who needed to adapt things to suit their medical condition. I worked out how to do the various leg stretches whilst sitting on the floor, with the aid of a stretch band, then taught the instructor so she could pass it on to anyone else who needed to know. Although I'm not sure she'll ever bother.

When there were more people than "stations", the instructor would add extra exercises until we had enough for one each. These additional ones were always walking exercises, so she didn't have to fetch additional kit. Those of us who couldn't walk well (including me on my crutches) were told to just sit out of those parts. Which seems to invalidate the whole idea of exercise sessions!

Several people started the program and dropped out after a few sessions, often after complaining to the rest of us about the instructor's lack of flexibility.

Those who stuck with it certainly benefitted from taking part. Unfortunately, it only lasts a few months and each person then has to either join the Leisure Centre or find another way to keep up their exercising. I object strongly to paying full-price for a gym membership where I'm not allowed or able to use much of the kit, so I choose to "work out" at home. I have a set of exercises that get done when I have the time and energy; so no exercise on days when I'm not feeling too good! I can't always do an exercise the way other people do, so I've adapted some to accommodate my limited fitness but give as much benefit as possible. I don't do much in the way of aerobic exercises, but I do a range of stretches, balances and some weight-training, too. Visitors have commented on the presence of dumbbells, gym ball, stretch bands, etc. in our lounge. It may be unorthodox, but if it helps me keep fit and flexible, it's got to be a good thing.

My favourite form of exercise is definitely swimming. I don't have the stamina I used to have and I can't swim for miles at a time. Neither is it practical for me to go to a swimming pool very often – especially given the way some people behave when they find a wheelchair left at the side of the pool. So I try to avoid sessions that are open to everyone.

I contacted our local pool:

"Hello. Can you tell me if you have a slot reserved for disabled people to swim?" I asked.

"No, we don't. There's no demand for it," she replied.

"Really? I'd have thought there were enough disabled people in town to make it worthwhile," I said.

"Well, we get two or three a week phoning."
"But there's no demand?"

Maybe I missed the point, but if a few people phone each week, doesn't that mean there's a demand for it? Maybe I should organise a wheel-in protest. We could all sit outside in our wheelchairs, wearing swimming costumes. I'm sure the local press would be interested. Ideally, I like to have a pool handy where I can swim a few lengths several times a day - so I'll just treat myself to swimming when I'm on holiday or staying in a hotel. Little and often is certainly the best way for me to keep fit.

With the advent of computer-based training systems, it's easier than ever for people to exercise in their own house. More and more disabled people are discovering the joys of a dance mat or a balance board, as well as those who have exercise bikes, walkers or rowing machines. As with any form of exercise, it's best to check that your doctor is happy for you to do it, especially before you spend any money!

Being at home all day could make anyone disabled, even if there was no problem with their mobility to start with. It's very easy to settle on the sofa, never walking further than the kettle or the bathroom. Keeping active helps to maintain a healthy weight, reduces the risk of further health problems and gives you something to do! Exercise is good for the mood as well as the muscles. Prescribed exercise schemes run in different parts of the UK (and maybe elsewhere). Or maybe your local leisure centre or gym has a "slot" for less-able people. It's worth asking around and taking advantage of whatever's out there.

The old saying applies very well to the human body – *use it or lose it!*

The Write Way

Although not strictly anything to do with chronic illness, I've been asked about writing in connection with disability so often that I thought it worth adding a couple of chapters on the subject. I only started writing when I finished full-time work years before I was ready to retire. Also, I find that many disabled people write or want to write – and they sometimes ask my advice on how to write or to get their work published. If you've ever wondered about this, then these chapters are for you.

My thinking, at the time I stopped work, was that writing was something I could do on days when I have the energy and leave alone when I wasn't well enough[3]. This has worked reasonably well in the years since then, although it can be frustrating when there's something in my head demanding to be written down and I don't have the energy to sit up and type. Incidentally – that's what I mean when I say writing. Typing. My handwriting was never exactly neat, and the MS has rendered it almost completely illegible.

So – how to write? It's quite simple, you just pick up a pen or a keyboard and get down to it. How to write well is much harder. There are many courses around on creative writing and I'd recommend any aspiring writer to check these out. Some are better than others, but you usually won't find out until you've actually forked out the

---

[3] At the time I made this decision, I never expected that my writing would take off the way that it has. Despite my limited energy, my writing has appeared in numerous magazines and I've won prizes in competitions. I may not be able to do it full-time, but that doesn't mean I do it badly!

cash – and cost is a significant factor for most of us. Check out your local colleges, magazines aimed at writers and search the internet for correspondence courses. Your local library may be able to help. Work out how much time you might be able to devote to your learning and decide what you want from a course. A few important points to consider:

- Do I get individual feedback from the tutor? (Absolutely essential. Comments from peers aren't likely to help much – how well could you advise someone else?)
- What sort(s) of writing does the course cover? "Creative Writing" is a big field and a course on poetry won't be very helpful if you're planning to produce a how-to guide on gardening for the disabled.
- Are there any guarantees? At least one correspondence course offers a refund of your fees if you haven't earned at least the same amount by the end of your studies with them.
- Is there a qualification at the end? Courses offered by colleges always offer some kind of certificate at the end of a successfully-completed course. Speaking personally, I'm not convinced there's much value in a creative writing qualification, unless you're planning to teach.

As mentioned above, these courses usually cost money, which may put many people off them, but it needn't. An aspiring writer can fund their "habit" by using their writing to earn as much as it costs. Start by looking at magazines you read. Do they have a letters page? What do they pay - £30? £50? Freebies? These small sums soon add up once you apply yourself. Put pen to paper and start sending off letters. The first few may not be accepted, but your newly-acquired writing skills will soon bring in the occasional cheque or package. There's a very nice DAB radio in my kitchen from just such an exercise.

There are a huge number of events and residential courses aimed at aspiring writers, from workshops at local libraries to weeks in sunnier countries. I'm a big fan of recreational education and have been to my fair share of them. Be aware that the quality varies tremendously, and the level of accessibility even more so. A few notes from my own experience:

- A Writer's Conference weekend where they couldn't provide accessible accommodation and I had to enlist other writers to help push my wheelchair up and down the hill between accommodation and conference centre.
- A weekend course where the staff would happily drive me between buildings, as the beautiful setting was too hilly for my wheelchair.
- A residential course where I was sent home early because I was being threatened by another course member – and they've been stalling for months over the promised refund.

I make a point of sending my comments on accessibility after attending one of these courses, with specific suggestions for how things could be improved, often at minimal cost. Sometimes a simple change to the wording of their advance information will make a big difference to the next person who's thinking of attending. These suggestions are rarely acted on, even when I've been asked to provide them. I have noticed that the organisers who take me up on my suggestions are the ones already trying to make their courses accessible. Others don't appear to pay any attention to simple ways they could improve. It's a shame, but that's life.

Many novice writers worry about their language skills. You don't have to use perfect spelling, grammar and punctuation to be a successful writer. If your story is good enough, the writing can be polished for you. There are online forums where people help each other out in this way – but you'll have to reciprocate. You can even pay someone to ghost you, but be warned – ghost writers cost money. I've done some ghosting and thoroughly enjoyed much of it – but I don't do it for free. There are plenty of reference books, but it's easier to look for an example in a novel you're reading! Don't let poor English stop you writing – but do the best you can and polish it up in the edit stages. Your grammar and spelling will improve as you practice.

There are three important steps to good writing. The first is to read. Lots! I always recommend that new writers read as much of their chosen genre as they can. You're not nicking plots or copying someone else's style, but you'll soak up the style of the genre. There's a big difference between the language used for romantic novels and the phrasing of crime stories. Read plenty and the style will become part of your writing. You'll find your own "voice" through experience, so don't worry you're nicking someone else's.

The next step is to write. I've lost count of the number of people who've told me they've got an idea for a bestseller, but haven't written a word yet. You can use whatever mechanism you prefer – many people write in longhand first and then type it onto a computer. I start at a keyboard. I never learnt to touch-type, but I'm a pretty fast two-fingers-on-each-hand typist now. The advantage of having my work in electronic form is that I can keep back-up copies and it's easy to edit.

The third step is to polish your writing. This is the stage that defines a *good* writer. I draw a similarity between writing and the visual arts. Many people think writing is like painting – that you start with a background setting, adding layers of plot and characters, drawing in the little details and adding more on top. I see it more in terms of sculpture. You start with a rough block of stone – your first draft; you then knock off big blocks of unnecessary waffle, gradually chipping off smaller pieces until you're finally down to something you can polish until it shines. I like this analogy because it makes the point that I spend more time editing than writing – and that it's hard work. Gene Fowler (an American journalist and author) famously said, *"Writing is easy. All you do is stare at a blank sheet of paper until drops of blood form on your forehead".* He's right – it is that easy.

You could ask your local library if they know of any writers' groups, but be warned. Many of these are more interested in socialising than in writing. Go along to a meeting or two and listen to what goes on. Are any of the members published? How good is their writing? What sort of comments do they make about each others' work? Does everyone get to read or is the meeting time dominated by one person who reads out 5,000 words of their latest never-to-be-polished book and won't allow anyone to suggest improvements? If your intention is to improve your writing then you need a group that will criticise and help you improve, whilst expecting you to learn how to do the same. Such groups are rarer than the social type – but they do exist.

If this chapter has struck a chord and you're fired up with a head full of ideas – then write them down. Your book will never happen if you don't start. So put pen to paper. Or fingers to keyboard. Or mouth to microphone and dictation software. Whichever you prefer. Start small – get a few letters published to boost your confidence and keep you going as you tackle something longer. Polish until your work shines and I look forward to seeing your name in print.

Publish and Don't be Damned

So you've written your book and you're wondering how to get it into print. The traditional routes into book publishing are well-known and there are some excellent, widely-available reference books. Check the shelves of your local library for recent editions of The Writers' and Artists' Yearbook or the Writers' Handbook, amongst others.

But submitting your work to a series of publishers and waiting for responses takes years, with no guarantee that the book will ever be printed.

Alternately, a growing number of companies offer to self-publish your work. For a fee. I don't call this self-publishing as it's under someone else's publishing company. If you want fifty copies of Grandad's memoirs printed for the family, this may be the way to go – but be warned, it's not cheap.

There are also services that offer a print-on-demand service where they hold your book electronically and print single copies when ordered. Expensive for your customers, but maybe the best option if you're only expecting to sell a limited number of copies.

So what about the middle ground? Technology has made it possible to print books quickly and cheaply from computer files that anyone familiar with a good-quality word processor can produce. Yes, you still pay upfront for the printing and binding, so it can be called vanity publishing. But the costs are reasonable enough that you may be able to make a profit from selling your work. Trust me, I've done it.

Naturally, this lower-cost option means more work for the writer who's decided to self-publish, but it's not as difficult as it might appear. Here is a list of steps that I follow, which I have provided to many other writers over the years. Please note that things may change between me writing this and you reading it. And please don't assume (as some writers have) that I'm offering to do the work for you. I've got my own writing to do...

After writing a book, the first step is to decide what you want to do with your work. *Is* it good enough to publish? Can you afford the printing costs up front (even if you later *make* money)? Who will buy your books? Are you prepared to make the effort to sell them? How many copies do you realistically expect to sell? Be honest with yourself, do the sums and decide which way to go.

When you're sure you want to publish and you've got a few hundred pounds you can invest in the venture, then you need to decide how you're going to sell them. If you're planning to supply them to bookshops, you will probably need an ISBN. (International Serial Book Number – this book is **978-0-9552602-3-0** – have a look on the back cover). These are sold by Neilsen UK ISBN Agency: http://www.isbn.nielsenbook.co.uk/ and a block of ten numbers (minimum purchase) will set you back £111.86 - but is enough for ten books! It will take a couple of weeks for your order to come through, so don't leave it until the last minute.

Once you've got your ISBN allocation, you need to send your data to Neilsen to set you up on their database. It's not difficult and their Help Desk staff are really friendly. Their database holds info about you as a publisher and about each book that you've published and retailers get their data from here. So once you register a new book, it will automatically appear on Amazon and in the stock catalogues of book shops everywhere. All of this takes time, so load your data once you know how big the book is going to be, etc – so that it's available online by the time you launch.

One of the hardest decisions is how much to charge for your book. Many bookshops won't stock your book unless the price is printed on the cover, so you can't leave it blank if you plan to sell through shops. Obviously, the more you charge, the faster you cover your costs. But the less you'll sell. And retailers will keep a percentage of the cover price when they sell one, sometimes as much as 65%. Yes, the shop keeps almost two-thirds of the money the customer pays! Find out how much you can expect to get from each sale and make sure you won't end up paying for someone to buy your book. Remember, it's easy to sell a book for less than the price on the cover but you won't get anywhere if you want to increase the price you charge!

Locating a printing company on the internet is easy. Finding a good one is a little more complicated. The printers I use are CPI Antony Rowe, in Eastbourne (who are extremely friendly and helpful), but there are others available. The market changes quickly and different printers will suit different needs, so make sure you're only paying for the services you need and shop around.

The printers will expect you to supply your book as two files – one holding the text of your book and one that's a picture of the cover. Simple versions of these can be produced by a good word processor package – you'll have to create them as .pdf files, which will be under "Save As" on the menu. Don't forget to set up the correct page size and layout. I'd recommend taking lots of backups as you work through this for the first time. It's easy to make a mistake and ruin the file you're working on until you've got the hang of it. A backup means you haven't lost anything!

Once your files are ready, send them to the printers. I use email, but you could send a CD-ROM by post or anything the printers will accept. Then it's simply a case of waiting for the books to arrive, paying for them and selling as many as possible!

You'll probably want to give a few complimentary copies to people who've helped with the book or who might promote it for you. Some self-publishers send copies of their book to large publishing companies, hoping to attract a contract for further work. It's worth a try, if you're prepared to give away a few extras. One word of warning – you'll need to be hard-hearted with the number of people who insist you should give them a free copy. I draw up a list in advance and stick to it, otherwise I'd never cover my costs!

As a publisher, you are obliged to supply at least one copy to the British Library – six if you want a copy in each of the depositories. But once it's been catalogued, you can go and "visit" it. The nice people at the Aberystwyth Depository tell me they get a steady stream of authors doing just that. You'll need to register with the library, so contact them in advance if you're planning to visit.

There are other formats you can publish in. Large print books are simple to produce, once you've got the files set up for the standard-size book, but it will cost more money. Audio books are increasingly popular but expensive to produce. Braille printing is a specialism in itself. If you're interested in pursuing any of these options, then contact the RNIB through http://www.rnib.org.uk/ for assistance. If you're thinking of recording a few chapters – perhaps for your own website – then I'd recommend using the best recording facilities you can afford and talking nicely to any friends you have who hold an Equity card. Or just a good, clear, speaking voice.

It's increasingly popular to publish books in a format that can be downloaded onto e-readers. This costs less than publishing on paper, but it doesn't appeal to everyone. Details on how to go about this are readily available on websites that offer the service. You can mix and match between the various formats, you don't have to stick to just one or follow the same route that I have.

Hopefully all your friends and family will be queuing up to buy a copy of your opus, but then it gets difficult. If your book is aimed at people with a particular interest, find an appropriate way to advertise to them. What about paying for a table at your local Christmas Fayre where you can sell signed copies face to face? Approach local bookshops – independents have more flexibility but the chain stores will stock self-published works if you can persuade them your work is up to scratch. Prepare a press release and contact your local media – newspapers love a local success story and you may be invited for an interview on radio. Try to come up with an original line, rather than just "local writer publishes first novel". Set up a website or advertise on social networking sites. There's a big world out there, and people love books!

If all of this looks daunting, remember that it can take years to get your book accepted by an established publishing house and they'll still expect *you* to do most of the marketing. And they keep most of the profit. But if you're convinced that your book is worth it, got for it, Dear Reader, and I wish you well. Send me a promo copy and I'll review it for you.

Learning for Life

Residential courses run by private companies and trusts of various kinds are also available; lasting anything from a weekend to a week or more. This level of immersion can be great, but also increases the impact of any problems.

The prospect of leaving your nicely-adapted home for a few days can be daunting. I always speak to someone on-site *before* I book; I ask a lot of questions and try to anticipate possible problems. I encourage them to tell me about difficulties other people have experienced and ask for their suggestions. I make a real nuisance of myself! As ever, the reaction and level of information varies. But there's one thing that has always proved true:

It's never as accessible as I've been told.

One course on a university campus turned out not to have any wheelchair accessible accommodation at all. They'd assumed that any ground floor room was suitable – despite outside steps and narrow doors. The shower had no seat and no room for my wheelchair. Good job it was only for a weekend!

The occasional venue offers a mobility scooter to make life easier for the less-mobile attendee. But older models often have a maximum weight of only 80 kg – 12½ stone in old money. They may not be well-maintained and never have a wheelchair carrier. In theory, a scooter would allow me to get around the campus and even find a little privacy –as other people might go for a walk. But when the scooter struggles to cope with steep paths and adverse cambers, it's wise to carry your mobile phone to call for help. I've taken my own off-road buggy on courses and love the freedom that gives me; I'm no longer reliant on other people's help to escape that single building.

Some venues are inherently difficult for those with limited mobility and I'm frequently excluded by poor accessibility. Once, assured the whole campus was accessible, I foolishly asked where the lift to the mezzanine area was. I've even had to pay extra for the only wheelchair-accessible room because it was en-suite, on a weekend where 30% of the activities were unreachable. Even when venues are accessible, a thoughtlessly-placed chair can be all it takes to prevent a wheelchair user reaching the area where people congregate. People who prefer to keep parts of the course exclusive – especially the social side – quickly realise how easy it is to block access in this way.

When there is designated accommodation for the less-mobile, the adaptations are limited – obstructions are common, alarm cords are rare. Picture the scene. It's 4 a.m. and you can't sleep. You want to call an ambulance; but your mobile has no coverage. There's a payphone on another floor, but people have complained about the noisy lift and you'd probably have to shift chairs to reach it. Are you well enough to move furniture as well as yourself? And are you prepared to wake everyone else?

The importance of staff's attitudes cannot be overestimated. One tutor was completely unfazed by my disability and remains one of my closest friends to this day. Another changed his one-to-one sessions to an upstairs room and "forgot" to join me in the coffee bar as he'd promised. Many fail to hide their unease; one visibly-uncomfortable tutor interrupted my 20-minute one-to-one session after 11 minutes, made his excuses and shooed me out. It's extremely rare for tutors to have had any disability awareness training and many prefer to simply ignore us - saying they'll "get back to you" and never doing so. Some think they're "doing the right thing", not realising they may be doing the exact opposite. Rarest of all are the people who ask what they can do and *check* whether their assumptions are correct.

Tutors don't realise how little is accessible to less-mobile participants. They'll state that they're available to chat at certain times, but they won't say where – because it's obvious to everyone. Well, everyone who can walk. Similarly, suggesting that delegates should speak to them at meals isn't helpful when their table is unreachable because of furniture or steps. Requests for a quiet chat are often ignored. If you get hold of a tutor, they will generally only be prepared to discuss your disability, asking for pointers on making the course more accessible. Socialising isn't an option. Everyone sees the disability, not the person.

Leper syndrome is as common on a course as anywhere else, and several days of carefully never touching a hand or reaching towards anyone is very wearing. But then you turn from the tutor who won't shake hands to the delegate who hugs you and thanks you for being an inspiration.

On one weekend conference, prizes were awarded after Sunday lunch. One was for "The Best Disabled Person" and it was explained that this had been awarded to the same person for several years, because she never complained about anything. I'd noticed the lady in question sitting on a bench for most of Saturday. She seemed thrilled to get the award and I wondered if it was the main reason she attended. Several delegates expressed their annoyance to me afterwards – but I doubt they told the organiser of their discomfort.

Some students resent what they see as the negative impact of having a wheelchair user on *their* course. One person on a recent course made it very clear that she begrudged the tutors switching rooms to make things easier for me. The same person complained that I'd been given a double room to myself (true but necessary – and how did she know?) and had been excused my share of kitchen duties (*not* true). The usual disability-envy problems are heightened by the close atmosphere of a residential course when everyone's feeling a long way from home and some are looking for scapegoats.

Bullies home in on a wheelchair as if there's a target painted on the back. Sometimes they claim they've got your best interests at heart; one student nagged me to wear shoes even in my wheelchair. She not only failed to convince me, but inspired me to knit some brightly patterned socks to wear on courses! Some people see me as a sucker who can be conned into taking their kitchen duty or swapping tutorials. Companies and charitable trusts are even less likely to require teaching qualifications than local authorities, so staff are neither trained nor inclined to deal with bullying. Coupled with the added opportunities of communal meals and shared accommodation, it's very easy for someone to make things very difficult. I've had things stolen and the sterile packaging of medical equipment opened. I've even had my wheelchair tampered with while I was out on a mobility scooter.

Food can be a major problem for those whose diet is restricted. Caterers often refuse to prepare individual dishes, so the choice is limited to "meat" or "vegetarian". It should be easier at smaller venues, especially when the students help in the kitchen, but sometimes people forget. Whether through ignorance or choice, people help themselves to the dish that's been prepared as your alternative and even serve inappropriate food onto your plate. No-one ever checks why someone is skipping meals. I always take a "snack stash" to fall back on.

It must be obvious when the person in the wheelchair is the only person missing from a group, but no-one passes on information that's been given to "everyone" – like a change of venue or time. Thus the disabled person is relegated to the last slot or misses out on opportunities. Even though I make a point of signing up for anything as quickly as I can, I'm often swapped with someone else or pushed out completely. Any attempt to address this is seen as being "needy" and rarely gets a better result than a figurative pat on the head.

It's important to make your own contribution. I *always* send a written report about accessibility issues afterwards. Good as well as bad. I detail improvements that can be made, sticking to practical suggestions and never blaming anyone. I include a paragraph that can be incorporated into their advance documentation to assist any future wheelchair users. I've offered to do formal site surveys for expenses only. I ask to speak to someone on the phone about the less-tangible problems, but no-one *ever* returns my calls. I've been told I'm being selfish to raise these things – even when I won't be going back and have no chance of benefitting myself.

To date, I don't know of *any* of my suggestions being taken up.

After all of the above, it's clear how difficult adult education courses can be for a mobility-impaired person. People with other disabilities talk of different problems – some worse than anything I've experienced. But I love education. I've learnt a lot on these courses, met many interesting people; made some useful contacts and even a close friend or two. Life is for learning and I intend to keep doing so as long as I can.

Local Learning

Another area of difficulty is adult education. I've studied on many courses over the years and met a variety of problems. Venues, courses and staff vary and it's important you're ready to make the extra effort, too.

For some reason, local colleges seem to be particularly bad at providing accessible venues. Even when an effort has been made, there often isn't the will to maintain accessibility. I appreciate that older buildings may be inaccessible and that retro-fitting ramps and lifts is expensive. But new campuses are still being built with limited access and simple measures are rarely taken, even when they'd cost nothing. A few examples, from a variety of colleges in different parts of the UK:

- The lift has been out of order since November and there is no money to fix it until the following academic year.
- The fold-out stair lift completely blocks the corridor for the 6 minutes it takes for you to get up or down. The lecture room is at the top, the only accessible toilet and the coffee bar are at the bottom and comfort breaks are a non-negotiable 15 minutes. Work it out!
- The campus has only three blue badge parking spaces, all occupied by cars without badges. You kick up a fuss and learn the cars all belong to able-bodied members of staff who use the spaces to stop non-disabled people parking there!
- The stair lift can only be operated by the trained member of staff who has the key – and they aren't available outside of office hours. Not even for an evening class.

- The day school at a leisure centre where the only accessible toilet is in the ladies' changing room in another building – I'm not sure where a disabled man is meant to go!
- The course where any activities that involve leaving the lecture room are scrapped, rather than addressing the inaccessible break-out room.

Another annoying aspect is that discounts are generally not offered for people with disabilities, - only pensioners, job seekers and those on a low income – even though a disabled person's involvement is restricted at least as much as theirs.

I tend to phone ahead of actually attending the course, to check about accessibility. Admittedly, I don't usually get much help. Sometimes the only person who can help isn't available and they never seem to return my calls. Or I'm told everything is accessible and left with a feeling that I'm talking to someone who doesn't care what they tell me. Not always, though. I've spoken to some very helpful people who genuinely want to know what I need. It's tremendously reassuring to hear comments like:

"I know the facilities aren't perfect – can you tell me afterwards if there's anything we can do to improve them?"

"I'm not sure if it's accessible all the way. I'll walk the route and get back to you."

"We'll swap rooms around to make it easier."

"Can you come ten minutes early for the first session? I'll take you round and check it's all okay."

As ever, the most helpful person is the one who asks, *listens* and acts.

Discrimination can go beyond the obvious area of accessibility. One course I attended with a local college ended with a formal appraisal of our work and the awarding of a qualification. At the first day school, one of the tutors made a point of chatting with me about access and related matters. She apologised for problems with room allocations which excluded me from certain activities and checked that I knew which way to go in the case of a fire alarm. Then she dropped the bombshell.

"We've had very few disabled people finishing this course."

"Really? I'd have thought it appealed more than the full-time alternatives," I replied.

"Most disabled people drop out before the end," she elaborated.

"I suppose that's not surprising, we're more likely to have difficulties that prevent us finishing," I answered.

"I shouldn't really tell you this," she leant closer and kept her voice low. "But no disabled person has ever got more than a C-grade for this course."

Well, it was nice to be warned, but what could I do about it? I completed the course, put my work in for assessment and got a C-grade, which I half-expected, although I believe my work merited more. The folder was missing several crucial pages when it came back, so there were gaps in my narrative and case studies missing, which would affect the quality of my work. I had double-checked that everything was included before delivering it to them, of course. You can't raise a case for discrimination without proof, and assessments are always subjective. But it would have been nice to feel I'd been assessed for my work, not my wheelchair.

Of course, it's not just the tutors who can discriminate against people with disabilities. Other students on a course can make life very uncomfortable. Fortunately, this usually manifests as an unwillingness to work with the disabled person, so the problem is largely self-resolving. The main problem area is when a bully decides to be difficult, but even this impact is diluted by the majority of people who go on a course to learn something.

Right at the start of this chapter, I mentioned the importance of being prepared to make the extra effort yourself. As well as the details mentioned above, there is one huge contribution that I make after a course. I *always* send a written report about any accessibility issues that arose. Good as well as bad. Wherever possible, I detail improvements that can be made. I stick to practical suggestions and avoid blaming anyone. I usually include a paragraph that can be incorporated into their documentation, to assist the next wheelchair user to come along. I've offered to do formal site surveys.

After all of the above, it's clear how difficult adult education courses can be for a mobility-impaired person. People with other disabilities talk of different problems – some worse than anything I've experienced. But I love education. I've learnt a lot on these courses, met many interesting people; made some useful contacts and even a close friend or two. I've just started a new course at a venue where I have to ride my buggy across the car park, over the playing field and round the back of the building to avoid a stair lift that's kept locked.

A little obstacle like that won't keep me from learning!

Afterword

And Finally

Dear Reader

we've reached the end of my little book. For me, this has been a long journey - many drops of blood over the years I've been writing it. It's been an emotional experience to revisit my experiences of disability; some happy memories, others less so. Looking back from a distance has left me better able to understand both what I was feeling at the time and why other people behaved the way they did. Writing as catharsis – it may be a cliché, but it does work.

I hope you've enjoyed reading along with me, that you've smiled at some points, perhaps understood your own experiences better while you've shared in mine. You won't agree with everything I've said and I'm sure there are areas I've omitted that you think I should have covered, but I hope you'll forgive me.

As I write this final chapter, I realise that I don't want the book to end. There are many more chapters I could write, so much more to say on the subject and I could keep editing and polishing for years. But it's already longer than originally planned and I've postponed publishing for too long. So the date is set and the book is going to the printers. I'm going to concentrate on fiction for a while – I want to write about characters other than myself!

Thank you all for coming on this journey with me. I hope I've told you something of value and I wish you much success whilst living with your own MonSters.

And always remember to look for the Rainbow.

Meg Kingston, Chepstow, October, 2010.